FOOD POISONING

AND

FOOD INFECTIONS

T0383899

FOOD POISONING

AND

FOOD INFECTIONS

BY

WILLIAM G. SAVAGE,

B.Sc., M.D. (Lond.), D.P.H.

COUNTY MEDICAL OFFICER OF HEALTH, SOMERSET; EXAMINER IN
STATE MEDICINE AND HYGIENE, LONDON UNIVERSITY; EXAMINER IN
PUBLIC HEALTH AND FORENSIC MEDICINE, BRISTOL UNIVERSITY

CAMBRIDGE
AT THE UNIVERSITY PRESS
1920

CAMBRIDGE
UNIVERSITY PRESS

University Printing House, Cambridge CB2 8BS, United Kingdom

Cambridge University Press is part of the University of Cambridge.

It furthers the University's mission by disseminating knowledge in the pursuit of
education, learning and research at the highest international levels of excellence.

www.cambridge.org
Information on this title: www.cambridge.org/9781107494879

© Cambridge University Press 1920

First published 1920
First paperback edition 2015

A catalogue record for this publication is available from the British Library

ISBN 978-1-107-49487-9 Paperback

EDITORS' PREFACE

IN view of the increasing importance of the study of public hygiene and the recognition by doctors, teachers, administrators and members of Public Health and Hygiene Committees alike that the *salus populi* must rest, in part at least, upon a scientific basis, the Syndics of the Cambridge University Press have decided to publish a series of volumes dealing with the various subjects connected with Public Health.

The books included in the Series present in a useful and handy form the knowledge now available in many branches of the subject. They are written by experts, and the authors are occupied, or have been occupied, either in investigations connected with the various themes or in their application and administration. They include the latest scientific and practical information offered in a manner which is not too technical. The bibliographies contain references to the literature of each subject which will ensure their utility to the specialist.

It has been the desire of the editors to arrange that the books should appeal to various classes of readers: and it is hoped that they will be useful to the medical profession at home and abroad, to bacteriologists and laboratory students, to municipal engineers and architects, to medical officers of health and sanitary inspectors and to teachers and administrators.

Many of the volumes will contain material which will be suggestive and instructive to members of Public Health and Hygiene Committees; and it is intended that they shall seek to influence the large body of educated and intelligent public opinion interested in the problems of public health.

AUTHOR'S PREFACE

FEW subjects are treated in textbooks both in such a hackneyed and in such an inaccurate fashion as food poisoning and food infections. The title "ptomaine poisoning" is maintained years after it has been proved that it is both inaccurate and misleading. Ptomaines are described in detail which have no bearing upon the question, organisms (such as *B. proteus* and *B. coli*) are accepted as the cause of attacks on the evidence of reports of outbreaks hoary with age, copied from textbook to textbook without any critical consideration as to how far they substantiate the claim, statements as to the distribution in nature of food poisoning organisms are repeated because some other textbook has admitted them and without any investigation as to their validity.

It follows naturally that, apart from those who have made a special study of the matter, the information as to the causation and nature of food poisoning outbreaks current amongst the medical profession generally, and even amongst those (such as Medical Officers of Health) who should be authorities, is to a considerable extent unsound and inaccurate. This has a very detrimental effect upon the scientific progress of the subject since it leads to outbreaks being ascribed to causes unwarranted by the facts and to inquiries into sources of infection being neglected in just those directions along which information would be most valuable. Anyone who has studied any considerable number of reports on food poisoning outbreaks will readily acquiesce in the truth of this statement.

To stimulate interest in the subject, indicate where exact knowledge is lacking and the directions where it may be sought, and to lay down lines of prevention are objects I have had in mind in writing this book.

Some of the views advanced are not in accord with those accepted in the textbooks but during the past fifteen years I have devoted much time to the investigation of the complex problems discussed and no current view is rejected and no new one advanced without the scientific data on both sides being fully stated.

The title is somewhat indefinite in scope and I have had to use my own judgment as to what to admit and what to reject as coming under it.

The subject treated from a narrower standpoint was dealt with by me in a special report to the Local Government Board in 1913, and I have to thank the Board and the Controller of His Majesty's Stationery Office, and in particular Sir Arthur Newsholme and Dr MacFadden, not only for their permission to make extensive use of the material in that report but for enabling me to bring my list of British outbreaks more up to date by kindly placing at my disposal particulars of a number of cases reported subsequent to 1912.

WILLIAM G. SAVAGE.

Weston-super-Mare.
October 1919.

CONTENTS

CHAPTER I

INTRODUCTORY AND HISTORICAL

The consumption of food, apart from the question of errors of quantity, may be a source of ill-health in a number of ways, the following being the most important:

(*a*) The food may be inherently poisonous. Noxious plants are well known, while animals, the flesh of which is poisonous, either always or at special times, are not uncommon.

(*b*) The food may be a cause of disease because it acts as a vehicle for the transmission of disease-producing bodies—of plant origin (such as ergot), of animal origin (such as the animal parasites), or of bacterial origin (anthrax, tubercle bacillus, etc.)—which are introduced with the food and which are directly derived from diseased plants or animals.

(*c*) The food may originate from healthy sources but subsequently become contaminated with bacteria pathogenic to man. The food may remain not visibly altered or may have undergone extensive decomposition changes.

(*d*) The food may be prejudicial because it has become admixed with bodies of a chemical nature which exert a harmful action upon the animal organism. Examples of such additions are chemicals added as food preservatives and poisonous metals derived from food containers or accidental admixture.

Admixture of food substitutes which irritate the alimentary tract to the extent of producing symptoms may possibly be grouped under this heading.

(*e*) The food may be so treated in preparation that valuable and essential substances have been removed, causing the so-called deficiency diseases.

(*f*) The food itself may be sound and uninfected with either harmful bacteria, parasites or chemicals and yet may originate illness in certain individuals owing to the existence of a special abnormal sensitiveness (idiosyncrasy conditions).

This is an extensive list and using the terms food poisoning

I

and food infections in their broadest meaning all might be so included. The title bacterial food infections excludes consideration of the animal parasites transmitted through food. Also the diseases induced by the removal of essential food constituents are negative rather than active in their origin and cannot be considered to come properly within the scope of the present volume. These deficiency diseases, as they are frequently called, include beri-beri, scurvy and probably pellagra, and are due to the diet being insufficient in certain essential substances known as vitamines, which are contained in the natural foodstuffs, but which may be removed in the course of preparation. They will not be further considered.

Common usage has given to the title of this volume a more restricted meaning and while this interpretation is one which cannot be defended as either entirely accurate or strictly scientific, yet it provides a convenient delimitation of an otherwise very scattered and far-embracing subject.

The infections induced in man by the consumption of meat from animals definitely ill with bacterial infections, such as anthrax or tuberculosis, and in which the like disease is set up in the persons infected, are true examples of bacterial food infections, but as they are fully dealt with in general and special textbooks they are only given comparatively brief consideration.

The cases in which the food merely acts as a vehicle for the transmission of the bacteria of well-known infectious diseases are conditions not generally understood when the above expressions are used although it is obviously impossible to set up a sharp scientific line of demarcation. A brief general discussion is all that is required therefore in explanation of these infections (Chapter II).

The remaining conditions are those which are usually specially understood by the terms food poisoning and food infections, and these are treated in considerable detail in subsequent chapters. It will be seen that they comprise:

  1. Inherently poisonous plants and animals.
  2. Foods only poisonous because of abnormal reactions of the individual.

3. Bacterial food infections causing more or less acute symptoms of poisoning.

4. Food poisoning cases from admixture with harmful chemical substances.

While the group due to admixture of chemicals is of great importance, the majority of the outbreaks and cases which are recognized as cases of food poisoning are undoubtedly bacterial in nature, and it is to this branch of the subject therefore that attention will mainly be given. The symptoms caused are due to the food being infected with bacteria which produce toxic products, either before or after ingestion, to which the symptoms are due. Under this heading is included those cases in which the food has undergone bacterial changes outside the body, of the nature of putrefaction, and those in which the specific bacteria have produced little or no visible changes, but exert their most characteristic activities after consumption.

Food poisoning conditions are frequently classified according to the vehicle of infection, those due to ordinary meat, shellfish, milk, cheese, ice-cream, sausages, fish, potatoes, etc., being separately described as if they had a separate and special causation. A few of these show special peculiarities with possibly a separate and peculiar etiology and so are more conveniently considered from this point of view, but apart from these such a classification is a most unscientific one and has nothing to recommend it. The vehicle of infection has little or nothing to do with the type of infection and the only scientific classification possible is one based upon the infecting agent.

The extent to which individuals are prejudicially infected through the agency of food cannot be estimated even approximately. The attacks may be so variable in severity, ranging from a trifling gastro-intestinal disturbance to severe symptoms dangerous to life itself and sometimes forfeiting it, may be so obscure and insidious in origin and so little anybody's business to investigate and record that it is quite impossible to statistically estimate their frequency. Most persons are attacked, at one time or another, with symptoms pointing with reasonable certainty to a derange-

ment of the alimentary tract set up by some article of food
eaten shortly before the illness. When these attacks involve
a number of persons there is more likelihood of their being
recognized as a food poisoning outbreak, but even the
majority of these pass unnoticed in the scientific journals or
in the daily press.

All that can be said is that attacks of illness from specific
contamination of the food are undoubtedly of considerable
frequency and that even extensive outbreaks are probably
far more prevalent than the published records of them would
lead anyone to believe.

Short historical account.

Food poisoning must be as old as man himself. In the
days of his dawning intelligence when driven by hunger or
the delights of the eye to experiment with strange foods he
no doubt learnt by bitter practical lessons that death and
illness lurked in many foods and by painful experience acquired a knowledge of good and evil as it applies to food.
In later times with more detailed knowledge as to foods
death still lurked in the pot but it was frequently enough a
deliberate death induced by malice, and the very widespread
institution in ancient historical times and in the Middle
Ages of official food tasters to king and princeling is a witness
of the prevalence of the practice of wilful food poisoning.
On the other hand in an age when sudden death was always
mysterious and suspect, food was no doubt frequently considered to be poisoned when it was not and death was due
to other causes. Over-indulgence in food was probably far
more frequently a cause of death than deliberate poisoning
and an instance such as the death of Henry I from lampreys
was more likely to be due to the surfeit of these fishes to
which it is ascribed in the history books than to any poisonous
qualities inherent in the lampreys, although it is a well-
recognized fact that under certain conditions lampreys exhibit poisonous properties.

"Death in the pot" still exists although man has catalogued
the poisonous plants and animals, scheduled and restricted

the sale of poisons and made gluttony unfashionable and an offence against taste. Now it takes other forms in large part due to the greed of man and his desire to acquire riches regardless of health considerations. Food is deliberately sophisticated, not in a spirit of vengeance but in one of greed or merely of callousness. Preservatives are sometimes necessary but are often added to conserve that which has become unfit or to keep in saleable condition for long periods what lack of cleanliness in preparation has imperilled. Animals are slaughtered "to save their lives," and to be sold as killed meat fit for food, while diseased meat is washed, doctored and disguised to take its place and obtain its price with the fresh and pure. Strict cleanliness in the preparation of all foods is not enforced and frequently is impossible under many of the prevailing conditions, in part because knowledge does not illumine the business and in part because cleanliness costs a little more. These are the forms that "death in the pot" takes to-day.

Many of the classical authors, such as Hippocrates, Horace and Ovid, refer to mushroom poisoning and some mention other poisonous foods. That food adulteration was practised in early times is clear from the importance given to it in many early enactments and the particulars mentioned by early writers. Wynter Blythe (*Foods, their Composition and Analysis*, 1903) quotes a number of interesting instances in which food was adulterated in Roman, Grecian and early English times.

The early conceptions of food poisoning were purely chemical in nature and this without invoking bacterial action upon the food to produce the chemical poisons. Albert von Haller was apparently the first to make any scientific studies upon the effects of putrid materials upon animals. He found that the injection of watery extracts of putrefying meat into the veins of various animals frequently produced death, while Gaspard in the early part of the nineteenth century carried on similar experiments.

In 1820 and 1822, Kerner published his papers upon poisonous sausages, ascribing the poisonous properties to a compound of sebasic acid and a volatile principle. We now know that these outbreaks were cases of botulism and due to a bacillus.

Later conceptions of food poisoning, and particularly of meat poisoning, were chiefly based upon the supposed relationship of the poisonous element to putrefactive decomposition of the food, and very numerous investigations were made along this line of inquiry.

Panum, in 1856, appears to have been the first to demonstrate that the poisonous qualities exhibited by putrid flesh were chemical in nature and not destroyed by boiling. Bergmann and Schmiedeberg, in 1868, obtained a highly toxic substance which they called "sepsin" from putrid yeast and from decomposing blood. After this discovery, other allied toxic bodies were discovered and extensively studied, and the whole group of basic substances with alkaloid characters were called *ptomaines* by Selmi. Selmi, however, did not himself succeed in isolating any of the putrefactive alkaloids, all his experiments being made with extracts, and Nencki, in 1876, was the first to isolate any of these bodies. Brieger (1882 to 1888) isolated and investigated a number of ptomaines.

Cadaverine was the first putrefactive alkaloid prepared by synthetic methods. This was done by Ladenburg in 1883, who determined its formula as pentamethylenediamine. Vaughan played an important part in the development of this side of the subject, and in 1884 isolated from cheese, which had caused poisonous symptoms, the body tyrotoxicon, a substance closely allied to the ptomaines.

The ptomaines, being bodies highly toxic to animals (when injected) and being obtained from putrefying meat, were at one time held to supply the cause and explanation of most, if not of all, cases of food poisoning and illness, and these outbreaks became fairly generally known, especially in this country, as cases of ptomaine poisoning. Indeed, at the present time, not only in popular estimation, but even amongst medical men and in scientific textbooks, this term is still largely retained, although, as will be shown later, there is no justification for its continued use.

It will be explained in Chapter VII that ptomaines differ

essentially from toxins in that the former are non-specific, while the latter are specific in that each is an intimate product of the bacterium which produces it.

The great strides now being made in Biological Chemistry have yielded much information as to the composition of the protein molecule and the different substances which result from its decomposition, and also as to how far these products are harmful and a possible cause of food poisoning.

While the ptomaine hypothesis largely held the field as the correct explanation of these outbreaks, another (a bacteriological) conception was gradually being evolved, the two hypotheses developing concurrently and being to some extent complementary to one another.

Bollinger, in 1876, in an important paper read at Dusseldorf, drew attention to the great importance of meat poisoning and to the fact that many outbreaks were associated with pyaemic and septicaemic conditions of the animals from which the food was obtained. He pointed out that the toxins of these diseases were not destroyed by cooking.

In a later paper, in 1880, Bollinger collected the literature of the subject and was able to emphasise further the relationship between human food poisoning outbreaks and septic, pyaemic and gastro-intestinal conditions in the animals whose flesh was consumed. The bacteriological proof of this relationship was not however forthcoming for a number of years.

Amongst the first bacteriological investigations on the subject were those of Klein, in 1880 for the Local Government Board, into the outbreak of food poisoning at Welbeck (Notts), due to eating infected ham. No definite proof was however adduced that the bacteria isolated had caused the disease.

The first important landmark in the bacteriological investigation of food poisoning outbreaks was the isolation by Gaertner in 1888 of *Bacillus enteritidis* from a meat poisoning outbreak at Frankenhausen. The bacillus was isolated both from the fatal case and from the organs of the cow, killed on account of enteritis, the consumption of whose meat caused the outbreak.

Since that date this bacillus, or closely allied forms, have been isolated from a very large number of outbreaks both in this country and abroad, and the etiological relationship has been firmly established. Indeed it is hardly too definite a statement to make that food poisoning of bacterial origin is very largely Gaertner group food poisoning and infection, and only in comparatively few cases are other bacilli associated etiologically.

The bacteriology of food poisoning also owes much to Van Ermengem. He investigated a number of outbreaks due to *B. enteritidis* and allied bacilli, while in particular, in 1896, he isolated and studied *B. botulinus*, the cause of an important group of food poisoning outbreaks (botulismus or sausage-poisoning), which were at one time especially numerous in Wurtemburg and other parts of South Germany. This form of food poisoning is unknown, or at least unrecognized, in this country. Although cases were reported in 1918 there was no real evidence that they were cases of botulism.

We owe an important further advance in the bacteriological study of food infections to Durham who demonstrated in 1898 that by the use of agglutination tests the bacilli isolated from food poisoning outbreaks, hitherto all indistinguishable, could be separated into at least two distinct groups. He also drew attention to the diagnostic value of the examination of the sera of patients suffering from food poisoning.

Independently, and nearly at the same time, De Nobele in Belgium came to similar conclusions.

On the epidemiological side this subject has received much attention from the Local Government Board. A very important summary of the then known etiological facts in relation to food poisoning was written in 1890 by Ballard (*Report of Medical Officer, Local Government Board*, 1890, p. 189), while an extended report on this subject, written by the writer, was issued in 1913 by the Local Government Board.

During the last twelve years or so a fresh impetus has been given to the subject and much additional light has been thrown upon it by the careful investigations which have been made as to the distribution of *B. enteritidis* and other bacilli of the Gaertner group in nature and their relationship to different diseases in man and animals.

Owing to the greater attention which the subject has received, especially during recent years, the number of recorded outbreaks of food poisoning is now considerable. Ostertag, in 1902, was able to collect records of eighty-five epidemics in the period 1880–1900, mostly from German sources, while the writer in the above-mentioned report was able to give an account of seventy-nine outbreaks in Great Britain and Ireland alone.

CHAPTER II

FOOD AS A VEHICLE FOR TRANSMITTING BACTERIAL DISEASES

THE subject of parasitic disease, apart from bacteria, is outside the scope of this volume and the present chapter is restricted to bacterial diseases. It deals on the one hand with the diseases of the domestic animals which are also harmful to man through their flesh or milk, and on the other with the general question of food acting as a vehicle for the transmission of infectious disease. Food poisoning outbreaks from specific bacteria or from putrefactive changes generally are dealt with in separate chapters.

Bacterial diseases of animals which may be transmitted to man by their flesh or milk.

The domestic animals, like man, suffer from many bacterial diseases. Some of these are peculiar to the lower animals and are not shared with man while others are common to both. As regards these diseases it does not follow that they are conveyed through food to man because they are common to both man and animals. Theoretically they may be, but probably few are so transmitted, owing to considerations which are dealt with later on.

Edelmann's *Meat Hygiene Textbook* (Mohler and Eichhorn's translation, 1916) gives the following list of infectious diseases of animals used for food transmissible to man: tuberculosis, para-tuberculosis (Johne's disease), pseudo-tuberculosis, actinomycosis, botryomycosis, anthrax, rabies, glanders, foot and mouth disease, variola, tetanus, malignant oedema, septicaemia, pyaemia and putrid intoxication. To this series must be added a few diseases such as Malta fever and some varieties of mastitis (garget) conveyed by milk.

The list is of formidable length but it is probably extremely rare if at all, for most of them, that these conditions are conveyed to man through eating infected meat and but few more from drinking infected milk.

Of these diseases tuberculosis is by far the most important and widespread, and tuberculous meat to a small degree and tuberculous milk to a considerable extent are important factors in keeping up the prevalence of these diseases, particularly in children. The bovine type of tubercle bacillus differs in certain characters from the human type but unfortunately possesses considerable virulence for man. The actual proportion of tuberculosis in man of bovine origin probably varies widely in different localities and is influenced by the habits of the inhabitants as regards the consumption of raw milk, etc., but very roughly it may be said that about 6 to 7 per cent. of deaths from tuberculosis are from bovine sources, nearly all being derived from tuberculous milk.

Anthrax, theoretically, may be spread from the milk or meat of infected animals, but it is probably very rarely so transmitted, the disease being acute in its course and the animal markedly ill and not likely to be sold for food. Infection from animals is usually by direct inoculation through the skin or by inhalation of the anthrax spores from infected wool or hair.

Foot and mouth disease may be transmitted to man through the milk of infected cows, but there is no evidence of its transmission by meat. The disease in man is of rare occurrence and usually is caused by direct inoculation.

Actinomycosis occurs fairly extensively in cattle, and recently Griffith (1915) has reported the presence of the specific organism in a large number of ox tongues from Argentina. The relationship between the human and bovine types has not been fully elucidated, but there appears to be no satisfactory evidence that this disease may be acquired by the ingestion of the milk or meat of infected animals. Our knowledge, however, requires extension particularly since this condition not very infrequently affects the udders of cows.

Botryomycosis is a not very accurately defined condition,

probably the result of infection with more than one species of microorganism. The writer is unaware of any evidence of cases of this disease transmitted to man by food.

For other diseases such as tetanus, glanders, rabies and variola (cow-pox and sheep-pox) which are met with in man the path of infection appears to be always, or almost always, by direct inoculation through the skin and not by way of the digestive tract.

The other diseases mentioned—malignant oedema, septic-aemia, pyaemia and putrid intoxication—stand in a rather separate category, since they are all conditions associated with rapid decomposition of the meat, and their liability to convey disease is less a question of the transmission of the bacterium responsible for the disease than of the secondary changes which the meat may undergo, either of the nature of putrefaction or of specific infection with one of the recognized food poisoning bacteria. Such conditions are therefore very wisely included amongst those which make meat unfit for food and cause its total condemnation.

The condition known as braxy, a disease of sheep fairly common in Scotland, possibly should be included in the same category. Food poisoning outbreaks in connection with sheep are very rare, so the following in Scotland is an interesting illustration recorded by Bryson (1907). In September, 1907, the weather being warm and sultry, a ploughman and other servants ate a meal consisting of broth and mutton. The latter was derived from a sheep, which four days earlier was found to be suffering from braxy and was killed in consequence. All the servants were attacked, but all except the ploughman quickly recovered after vomiting. In his case the symptoms came on 2–3 hours after the consumption of the food, being the usual ones of abdominal pain, vomiting, cramps in the extremities, and foul evacuations. He also suffered from bradycardia. The report is not very definite but apparently there was no evidence of obtrusive decomposition of the meat. The report throws no light on the real cause of the food poisoning, but no doubt the condition of the animal predisposed the meat to infection with Gaertner or other bacilli, although of course the condition in the sheep may have been due to infection with these bacilli. It can hardly be accepted that the condition of braxy was the cause of the outbreak.

In addition to the above-mentioned diseases there are two conditions spread by milk but not by meat. One is Malta fever, the specific organism of which, *Micrococcus melitensis*, is frequently found in goat's milk in Malta and other affected places, goat's milk being a very common vehicle for the transmission of the disease. This disease may also affect cows and be spread by cow's milk, but the writer has been unable to trace specific instances. The other condition is mastitis in cows, an inflammatory disease due to various organisms, some of which are pathogenic to man and which are capable, when transmitted by milk, of causing widespread outbreaks of sore throat and other septic conditions in man.

(For an account of this condition and also of outbreaks caused see the author's book, *Milk and the Public Health*, 1912, pp. 91–100 and 105–111.)

It will be obvious from the above remarks that, apart from a few diseases transmitted by milk, tuberculosis, diseases caused by bacilli of the Gaertner group and possibly local and general septic conditions, diseases of animals are not commonly transmitted to man through flesh derived from animals suffering from these complaints. Many common animal diseases which have not been mentioned, such as swine erysipelas, swine plague, blackleg, cattle pleuropneumonia, rinderpest, etc., are not, so far as is known, transmissible to man.

Food as a passive vehicle for the transmission of infectious disease.

The extent to which food acts as a passive vehicle for the transmission of infectious diseases depends upon a number of different factors, of which the most important are the nature of the food, the opportunities for infection and the degree to which sterilization or partial sterilization is practised before consumption.

Meat in its various forms and milk furnish bacteria with

abundant nutriment and are on this account particularly liable to act as vehicles, since the element of dosage enters to a considerable extent into the question of infection. When these foods are infected with pathogenic bacilli the latter are likely to multiply, become very abundant and be distributed over or through a good part of the food. Other foods, such as bread or cereals, are much less likely to transmit infection, as even if specifically contaminated little or no multiplication of such bacteria will take place. Vegetables occupy an intermediate position in this connection, but some such as watercress, which are eaten raw, are liable to carry infection.

Opportunities for infection vary greatly according to the foodstuff and the amount and kind of handling before being eaten. Certain foods, for example, are obtained from sources which are liable to be contaminated with sewage. Oysters, cockles and mussels, amongst shell fish, and watercress may all be contaminated from such material and typhoid fever has frequently been spread in this way. For other foods the chief danger lies in contamination with pathogenic bacteria during their preparation for sale. Meat, for instance, is liable to be splashed with the excreta of other animals or to be contaminated by dirty hands and instruments. For other foods the risk of their conveying disease is largely one of dirty and careless handling, and if the food handlers suffer from an infectious disease, or are carriers of the bacilli of such diseases, widespread infection may result. Milk and milk-containing foods, such as ice-cream, are liable to convey disease, either from diseased animals, carelessness in preparation or neglect in distribution.

The degree to which food is sterilized before consumption is of great importance as regards its serving as a vehicle of infection. Foods, such as oysters, mussels and ice-cream, which are eaten raw, have over and over again been convicted of spreading outbreaks of acute infectious disease. Other foods eaten raw, such as watercress and other vegetables, are only less liable because their opportunities to become infected are so much less. Others again, such as cockles and fried fish, which receive some cooking, but often of an ineffective character, also may serve to spread infectious disease. When cooked food is found to be the vehicle of spread it* almost invariably is so because the cooking has been inadequate to destroy pathogenic bacteria or more commonly because infection results after cooking and before consumption.

It may be mentioned that infection of food with pathogenic bacteria after cooking is more dangerous than if no heating had taken place. Many bacteria are mutually inimical and the hardier saprophytic types frequently serve a useful function by making the conditions of viability and growth difficult for the pathogenic types. When the former are destroyed by cooking this restraining influence is removed and the multiplication of any pathogenic bacteria which may gain access is likely to continue unrestrained. This fact constitutes one of the dangers of partially or wholly sterilized foods, such as brawn or pasteurized milk.

Cooking to be efficient must be sufficient to kill any pathogenic bacteria which may be present in any part of the food. It involves therefore two points: the actual temperature reached and the degree or rate of heat penetration. Meat is of particular importance in connection with food poisoning outbreaks so that some particulars of temperatures reached in cooking may be of interest.

Temperatures reached in cooking food.

A considerable number of the experiments upon this point have been carried out in Germany in connection with the problem of the destruction of trichinae in flesh. Küchenmeister with fairly large pieces of meat cooked in the ordinary way obtained the following average results, reached throughout the whole piece: broiled flesh 60° C., boiled beef 87·5° C., grilled beefsteak 56–57° C., roast pork (middle of joint) 65° C. He found that large joints required boiling for several hours for the interior to reach a temperature of 77–80° C. Meat is a poor conductor of heat. Perroncito carried out a number of experiments of which the following may be mentioned. The centre of a piece of beef (8 × 10 cm.) placed and kept in boiling water was only 47° C. after twenty and only

68–70° C. after thirty-five minutes. A ham of about six kilos weight was placed in cold water which was raised to boiling point. The water boiled when the interior of the ham was 25° C., after thirty-five minutes it was 35° to 40° C., and after two hours the temperatures in different parts of the interior were 46°, 55°, 58°, 62°, 64° and 67° C. A ham of about eight kilos treated in the same way only showed an interior temperature of 44·5° C. after 2½ hours, while after 3½ hours the temperatures varied from 62–84° C. in different parts.

Rupprecht found that boiling for forty-five minutes, as practised in Saxony, did not produce a higher temperature than 75° C., and this only in thin pieces of meat. He found that the interior temperature of a rapidly roasted sausage was only 28·7° C. Wolffhügel and Hueppe found that it was necessary to prolong the cooking of a leg of veal for 3½ hours at 101° C. for the temperature of the deep parts to reach 71–89° C. In another experiment a smoked ham of 4·5 kilog. weight (about 10 lbs.), 36 cm. long, 22 cm. wide and 10 cm. thick, was boiled in a cooking vessel in salt water for four hours at a maximum temperature of 102° C. The thermo-meter indicated temperatures of 75°, 77° and 78° C. in the centre of the meat.

Petri also tested the penetration of heat into large pieces of meat and found that even after 3½ hours' cooking the temperature of the interior may be only 84° C. or less.

These experiments demonstrate the fact that meat is a poor conductor of heat and that the temperatures reached by the interior of meat subjected to fairly complete cooking may be far below the temperature necessary to kill harmful bacteria. It will be shown later on that a large proportion of food poisoning outbreaks are associated with prepared foods, such as meat-pies, brawn, canned meat and the like, and it is of importance to note that the temperatures reached in the cooking of these articles may be quite insufficient to sterilize the food or even to kill such pathogenic bacteria as B. typhosus, B. paratyphosus B or the food poisoning bacilli, which are destroyed at comparatively low temperatures. A few examples may be mentioned.

In connection with the Derby food poisoning outbreak, Delépine and Howarth carried out some experiments upon the temperature reached in baking meat pies. They noted:

(a) The temperature of the centre of a pie said to be underbaked, but having all the external appearances of being well baked, may not exceed 47·2° C.

(b) The temperature of the centre of a pie obviously over-baked, and acknowledged to be so, had not reached beyond 86·6° C.

(c) There was a difference of several degrees between the temperature of various pies.

As Delépine points out, a batch of pies prepared in a hurry might be so cooked that bacteria might continue to grow in their centre during the greater part of their stay in the oven, and the bacteria would certainly not be killed.

The experiments of Beveridge and Fawcus (1908) upon the penetration of heat into the substance of meat in tins are of considerable interest.

They found that when a tin was simply boiled in water, the temperature of the centre of the meat did not reach 100° C. even at the end of five hours.

With higher temperatures the following results were recorded:

Outside Temperature	Size of Tin	Time taken by Central Thermometer to		Number of Experiments
		Reach 100° C.	Reach 105° C.	
107° C.	1 lb.	58 min.	80 min.	Average of 5
107° C.	2 lbs.	95 ,,	123 ,,	,, 5
120° C.	1 lb.	22 ,,	27·4 ,,	,, 5
120° C.	2 lbs.	28 ,,	36·2 ,,	,, 5
130° C.	2 lbs.	17 ,,	22 ,,	,, 2

With the ordinary large 6 lb. tins the rate and time of heat penetration would be much longer.

These experiments illustrate the ease with which the toxins of Gaertner group bacilli may escape destruction in tins of meat insufficiently heated.

It is not only meat foods which may spread infection and which may fail to be sterilized by cooking. Sawyer (1914), for example, records an interesting experiment with spaghetti, a substance which when made by a certain typhoid carrier caused an epidemic of typhoid fever involving ninety-three persons who consumed this food. Laboratory experiments showed that Spanish spaghetti artificially infected with typhoid bacilli and made exactly as the carrier made it and cooked in a hot air sterilizer until the surface was dark brown and it appeared overcooked, failed to be sterilized and thermometer readings showed that the interior did not reach even a pasteurizing temperature. Cultures from the surface yielded no typhoid bacilli and only a few half-an-inch below the surface, but cultures from a depth of two-and-a-half inches showed abundant colonies of this organism. The cooking of this food in this outbreak merely served to incubate and multiply the bacilli.

Milk as a vehicle of spread.

As regards different foods milk stands on a rather separate footing and merits individual mention. Certain considerations make it especially liable to convey infection.

(a)   It is commonly consumed raw or with inadequate cooking.

(b)   It is a particularly suitable nutrient medium for bacteria, so that those which gain access tend to multiply enormously, while milk being liquid they diffuse through the whole amount.

(c)   It is largely a food for children who are especially susceptible to infectious diseases.

(d)   It is a food which is extensively handled, thus giving abundant opportunities for infection, while the prevailing conditions under which it is collected and distributed are preeminently unsatisfactory.

(e)   It is derived from an animal which may herself be diseased and in that way supply milk already infected with pathogenic bacteria.

In view of these facts it is not surprising that outbreaks of disease spread by milk are frequent and widespread. The chief diseases so spread are tuberculosis, diphtheria, scarlet fever, typhoid fever, para-typhoid fever, sore throat, diarrhoea and gastro-enteritis, food poisoning. Cholera, Malta

fever, dysentery and other diseases not common in this
country may also be transmitted by milk.

Tuberculosis, sore throat outbreaks and Malta fever may
be derived from a diseased animal but all the others, and
these conditions sometimes, are nearly always spread by
specific contamination of the milk from human sources.
Such infection may be direct or indirect. In the former
method the milk handler is either an actual sufferer from the
infectious disease or a carrier of the specific organism. In
the latter the source of infection may be from infected
clothing or conveyed by infected water, dust, flies, etc.

The infectious diseases spread by food.

Apart from milk, foods do not usually act as vehicles of
transmission for many diseases and in this country they are
chiefly typhoid and para-typhoid fevers, tuberculosis, outbreaks of food poisoning and possible epidemic diarrhoea.
Other important conditions so spread, but rare in this
country, are cholera and dysentery.

Diphtheria outbreaks spread by food other than milk, or
milk products, are almost unknown, but Sobernheim and
Nagel (1918) have recently recorded an outbreak of eighty-
one cases in a Berlin garrison in which the vehicle of infection
was food infected from diphtheria cases or carriers. The
epidemiological facts definitely implicated the food from
the central kitchen as the vehicle, but the exact article of
food which was specifically infected could not be determined,
but it was probably a herring salad.

Typhoid fever is the most important condition so spread
and may be taken as an illustration. This disease is liable
to be transmitted in this way because, as is well known, a
proportion of recovered cases harbour the bacilli in their
bodies for long periods, not infrequently extending to many
years, excreting the bacilli intermittently in their urine and
faeces. If such persons are employed to handle food they may
readily infect it and cause outbreaks of typhoid fever. Such
outbreaks have been most commonly recognized in institu-
tions (probably, however, only from the better methods
employed to detect them) and the track of the carrier from

one institution to another can be traced by the crops of cases they infect. Outbreaks of this sort are not usually explosive, but generally creeping in character, since the opportunities to infect the food are intermittent and subject to many checks, while the chances of survival of the bacilli are sometimes precarious, at others favourable.

Milk is probably the commonest food to be infected in this way, but many other foods, such as meat, potatoes, bread, have been suspected or proved to be the vehicle of distribution. The career of the famous "Typhoid Mary" may be given as a good illustration of a chronic typhoid carrier acting as a food handler. She was a cook and was responsible for no less than twenty-six cases in seven different families. The final outbreak which led to the recognition of her baneful influence was in 1907 when two cases of typhoid fever occurred in the family where she served as cook and which took place two months after her arrival. Gaps in her history could not be traced but at least the following cases resulted in places where she was a cook: one case in 1901, one case in a second family in 1901, nine cases in another family in 1902, four in another in 1904, six cases in one family in the summer of 1906, and one in another family in the autumn of the same year.

Another interesting example reported by Niven in 1908 is Mrs W., who kept lodgers and did her own housework. No less than seven lodgers at different times between 1898 and 1908 contracted typhoid fever, while this woman in November, 1908, was found to have typhoid bacilli in both faeces and urine.

A number of other illustrations are given by Ledingham in his work on typhoid fever carriers.

Explosive outbreaks may be spread by infection of the food by a carrier, as in the outbreak mentioned above when ninety-three persons contracted typhoid fever from spaghetti, but are more frequently associated with contamination of the food with typhoid bacilli from sewage pollution. Many typhoid fever outbreaks from oysters have been caused in this way.

As a typical example may be instanced the outbreaks of

typhoid fever at Winchester and Southampton in 1902, following the Mayoral banquets on November 10th in these towns (Bulstrode, 1903). At the Winchester banquet there were 134 guests of whom nine contracted enteric fever and also one waiter. At the Southampton banquet there were 132 guests with ten cases and also one attendant. In both cases a number of the guests (forty-four at Southampton) suffered from gastro-enteritis of varying degrees of severity. By careful inquiry Bulstrode showed that the only item taken at the banquets capable of explaining the outbreaks were the oysters. Both lots of oysters were from the same source and were consumed in the two towns on the same day, while a number of other cases in other towns were shown to be due to oysters obtained from the same source and also consumed the same day. The oysters were derived from beds at Emsworth, which seven years previously Bulstrode had reported as liable to gross pollution. The oysters were laid down within a few yards of the main sewer of the town, one in which cases of typhoid fever had been unduly prevalent for years and in which several cases occurred shortly before the outbreak.

General conclusions.

From the above considerations it is possible to draw some broad general conclusions in regard to the transmission of infectious diseases by food.

1. In view of the many sources of possible infection of foodstuffs with pathogenic bacteria, there is always some risk, and as regards certain foods considerable risk, of their acting as vehicles for the transmission of infectious disease, if they are consumed in the raw state. Incomplete as is the protection afforded by cooking it is yet very considerable, and to realize this we have only to contrast the numerous outbreaks spread by milk and shell fish with the rarity of those associated with food habitually eaten cooked. It follows that foods eaten raw require special supervision in their preparation and transmission. In several places, such as Southend, the installation of efficient methods of cooking

cockles, replacing the previous haphazard and inadequate procedure, has resulted in a marked fall in the number of cases of typhoid fever.

2. Special supervision is required over those whose business it is to handle food. A chronic typhoid carrier is for the most part only a public menace when a food handler. This aspect of the subject has received very inadequate legal consideration in this country and there are no enactments which give effective powers to deal with this class of persons. The following may be mentioned in illustration. The writer recently investigated a small outbreak of six cases of typhoid fever in a small town, all within a short period of one another, and all with a common milk supply. Suspicion pointed to the milk purveyor himself, especially as a history of an obscure illness some years earlier was forthcoming. A sample of his blood, secured with difficulty, showed a positive Widal reaction. After much persuasion a sample of his excreta was obtained, but when this was negative no efforts were successful in obtaining a second. No further cases developed and the matter had to be left (particularly in view of the insufficiency of proof) as there were no legal powers to prevent this man continuing to milk his cows and distribute his milk.

The Department of Health of New York City in 1915 inaugurated detailed medical and pathological examinations of the cooks and waiters in a number of the hotels and restaurants of the city. A considerable number of typhoid carriers and infectious cases of syphilis, tuberculosis, etc., were detected in this way.

3. General cleanliness in the manufacture, preparation for sale, and distribution of food is of the utmost importance. Strict cleanliness and care in preparation will obviate many of the dangers of food acting as a vehicle of infection, while these precautions are even more necessary for foods which are liable to imperfect cooking or some degree of heating and are not consumed for some time. Ice-cream, pasteurized milk and some forms of made food come under this category. This aspect of the question is dealt with more in detail in Chapter XIII.

REFERENCES.

Beveridge and Fawcus (1908). *Journ. Royal Army Med. Corps,* x. 315.

Bryson (1907). *Brit. Med. Journ.* II. 1710.

Bulstrode (1903). *Report* to L. G. B. on oyster-borne enteric fever at Winchester and Southampton.

Edelmann (1916). *Meat Hygiene Textbook* (Mohler and Eichhorn's translation).

Griffith (1915). *Report* to L. G. B. Food Reports, No. 23.

Howarth and Delépine (1902). *Special Report on Outbreak of Food Poisoning in Derby.*

Savage (1912). *Milk and the Public Health* (Macmillan and Co.), pp. 91, 105, etc.

Sawyer (1914). *Journ. Am. Med. Assoc.* LXIII. 1537.

Sobernheim and Nagel (1918). *Berl. klin. Woch.* LV. 761.

CHAPTER III

FOODS INHERENTLY POISONOUS

THE rest of the book deals with foods which in themselves are sound and harmless, but which become poisonous or infective on account of secondary changes, either through the food acting as a nidus for bacterial growth or through contamination with chemical poisons. The present chapter deals with foods, both animal and vegetable, which in their natural state are poisonous to man.

Animals poisonous when eaten.

There are a good many animals which produce poisonous secretions as part of their defence against a hostile world, or utilize them as a means of killing their food, but such animals do not properly come under the above heading. Well-known examples are the poisonous snakes, certain fish, such as the sea-weaver, members of the scorpion family and a considerable number of insects. Their action is produced by injection into the tissues and such poisons are entirely or very largely inoperative when introduced by the mouth. These animals can be eaten without risk of poisoning.

The number of animals the flesh of which is inherently poisonous when eaten is small and, as will be shown later on, only a small proportion are poisonous at all seasons. In some cases—particularly as regards shellfish and some fish—the food is said to be poisonous at some seasons and under certain conditions, but these cases do not really come into the above category since they are not inherently harmful, but become poisonous on account of bacterial changes which they undergo associated with their environment. They are, therefore, dealt with in other chapters. Indeed the only animals of importance which remain are certain species of fishes with possibly a few poisonous shell fish.

Poisonous fish. Many fish, especially those native to tropical waters, develop poisonous bodies of the nature of toxins very rapidly after death, so that their consumption, even a few hours after death, gives rise to symptoms of poisoning, although such fish are quite harmless and wholesome if consumed perfectly fresh. Apart from these there are certain fish whose bodies, even when alive, contain toxic substances of great potency.

Of these fish by far the most important is the family of the Tetrodontidae. This family—the puffers, balloon fish, globe fish—comprises a number of poisonous species, including the well-known Japanese Fugu, which has a very large number of deaths to its credit. Faust (1906), for example, says that in the years 1885 to 1892 there were recorded in Japan 933 cases of poisoning from this cause, 681 (73 per cent.) of which were fatal. This family of fishes is widely distributed along the coasts of Japan, China, East Indies and Africa.

Poisoning from these fishes is very acute with rapid onset of symptoms. Savtschenko (1886) divides the cases into two groups, the choleriform and the gastro-intestinal. In the former the whole duration may be only from ten to twenty minutes to a few hours with very rapid onset of abdominal pains, great distress, prostration, collapse, diarrhoea, vomiting, cramps in the limbs, with death from respiratory or cardiac paralysis. The symptoms in the gastro-intestinal type approximate to those met with in ordinary food poisoning outbreaks.

The nature and distribution of the poison has been carefully studied by Takahashi and Inoko (1890), Miura and Takesaki (1890), Tahara (1890, 1911), and others.

These investigators found that the poison is mainly or entirely contained in the ripe ovaries (roe), alcoholic extracts from the other organs giving rise to no symptoms in rabbits. Tahara isolated from the ovaries two poisonous bases but in a later paper (1911) isolated tetrodotoxin from the roe as probably the only poisonous substance. He obtained it in the form of a white very hygroscopic powder readily soluble in water and with a lethal dose equal to about four mgrm. per one kilogrm. of body weight. It is neither an alkaloid nor a protein.

The concentration of the poison in the reproductive organs explains the facts mentioned by earlier observers, for example, as recorded by Günther (1880), that "the poisonous properties of these fishes vary much as regards intensity, only certain individuals of a species, or individuals from a certain locality, or caught at a certain time of the year being dangerous."

Günther mentions a number of other poisonous fishes including some varieties of herring (*Clupea thrissa, Clupea venenosa*), tunny fish, file fishes, etc., while he quotes Poey as enumerating not less than seventy-two different kinds from Cuba.

According to Schmidt a number of members of the sturgeon tribe are poisonous, the poison being confined to certain parts of the fish.

The barbel (*Barbus fluviatilis*) has been particularly credited by older writers with causing poisonous symptoms (barb-cholera). The roe appears to be the only part which is poisonous. Hesse in 1835 carried out over 110 experiments upon men with roes from barbel. In sixty-seven no symptoms were caused, while in forty-three some illness ensued, but this was mostly confined to abdominal pain or diarrhoea and in only two were cholera-like symptoms produced. No fatal cases have ever been reported.

Jordan states that the flesh of the Greenland shark possesses poisonous qualities for dogs and produces a kind of intoxication in these animals.

While a number of European fish are reputed to be poisonous at certain seasons of the year (particularly as regards certain parts of the fish), such as the barbel, sturgeon, carp, bream and one variety of perch (*Perca venosa*), it remains true generally that these poisonous fish are chiefly found in tropical waters. Very little accurate scientific work appears to have been done upon the exact cause of the poisoning properties of these fishes. The older writers lay stress not merely upon the fact that certain parts only are sometimes poisonous (chiefly the roe), but trace a relationship to the kind of food consumed. Thus Günther states that in the West Indies it has been ascertained that all the fishes living and feeding on certain coral banks are poisonous and suggests that they acquire this noxious quality from their food which consists of corals, mollusks and crustacea. The poisonous herrings are said to be toxic only when they have been feeding on certain special kinds of food. Mitchell (1900) states that in 1842 all the members of a family in Toulouse were poisoned by eating a dish of snails collected from a poisonous shrub (*Cariaria myrtifolia*).

More exact scientific investigation is required upon all these matters.

Poisonous plants and fungi.

The members of the vegetable kingdom which are poisonous and give rise to illness when eaten may be divided into three groups: those belonging to the flowering plants, the poisonous fungi, and certain special parasitic vegetable growths.

Poisonous flowering plants.

It is well known that there is a large number of plants all or parts of which are poisonous when eaten, but fortunately the majority of them are either not very common or not attractive as food and actual cases of illness from this cause rarely occur, and are mostly confined to children eating poisonous berries. Amongst the best known of such plants are the deadly nightshade, henbane, spotted and other varieties of hemlock, foxglove, hellebore, monkshood, laburnum, bryony, yew, tansy and pennyroyal. These plants owe their harmful properties to poisonous chemical substances, for the most part alkaloids, of which strychnine, atropine, conine and aconite are well-known examples. The symptoms vary according to the nature of the chemical active principles and these and other particulars are set out in detail in textbooks on Toxicology.

Although a few of them, e.g. water hemlock, which has been eaten in mistake for parsnips and for celery, are eaten in mistake for edible foods, these accidents are rare, so these conditions hardly come under the category of food poisoning and do not require further consideration here.

In this connection it may be mentioned that milk is said occasionally to have produced gastro-intestinal symptoms due to the consumption by the cow of certain poisonous plants, such as poisonous ivy (*Rhus toxicodendron*) or even the leaves of the common artichoke.

According to Müller the milk of goats which have eaten *Colchicum autumnale* has caused the poisoning of infants.

Poisonous fungi.

Poisoning by fungi usually results when certain noxious varieties are mistaken for edible kinds and are eaten as food. This condition therefore properly comes under the designation of food poisoning.

Cooke, writing in 1894, states that the number of species of poisonous fungi found in this country is comparatively small and with knowledge and experience the list is gradually being reduced.

In this country *Agaricus campestris* (the common mushroom) and, to a lesser extent, *Agaricus oreades*, are the only fungi eaten, but a considerably wider selection is made on the continent. Cases of poisoning appear to be most numerous in the United States of America, probably due to the large influx of a mushroom eating population from Southern Europe liable to confuse poisonous American varieties with rather similar kinds which are eaten without harm in their native lands. In illustration of this frequency it may be stated that Jordan (1917) mentions that in the vicinity of New York City there were twenty-two deaths from mushroom poisoning in one ten-day period (September, 1911) following heavy rains. The question of mushroom poisoning has naturally received special attention in America and we owe much of our recently acquired knowledge as to the nature of the poisons concerned to Ford and his fellow-workers in that country.

The fungi chiefly responsible for poisoning cases are *Amanita muscaria* (the fly fungus) and *Amanita phalloides* (death cup), but a large number of other fungi have been shown to possess poisonous properties: Cooke mentions twenty-two poisonous species in this country.

The symptoms of poisoning may be nervous or gastro-intestinal in type or more commonly a mixture of both. Common nervous symptoms are muscular twitchings extending to tetanic spasms or even general convulsions, disorders of vision and of the other special senses, somnolence and coma. The gastro-intestinal symptoms are the usual ones of nausea, vomiting and diarrhoea, with great thirst and prostration. The body is cold with weak quick pulse and laboured respiration.

McIlvaine (1912) experimented on himself with pieces of *Amanita muscaria*, the size of a hazel nut, and found that it produced vertigo, nausea, pallor, exaggeration of vision, and respiratory distress, the effects passing off in two hours leaving severe headache.

The poisonous properties of these fungi are all chemical in nature, although not the same for all the different species, and the degree and severity of the symptoms are proportional to the quantity of poison taken. There is not much evidence of idiosyncrasy in individuals and the well-known variability of toxicity of different plants of the same species can probably be explained on other grounds.

Ford (1910–11) divides the poisonous fungi into three groups:

A. Those containing poisons acting on the nerve centres, e.g. *Amanita muscaria.*

B. Those producing degenerative changes in the internal organs, e.g. *Amanita phalloides, Amanita verna,* etc.

C. Those causing gastro-intestinal disturbances of a more or less violent character, e.g. *Lactarius torminosus, Clitocybe illudens, Entoloma sinuatum,* etc.

From *Amanita muscaria* the substance muscarine has been isolated and studied in a pure condition by Schmiedeberg and Koppe. Although muscarine is a powerful poison the symptoms it produces in the human subject are not identical with those produced by this type of mushroom poisoning. Also an infusion of the fresh fungus is very poisonous to flies while muscarine itself is harmless to those insects. While, therefore, it is reasonable to assume that muscarine plays a large part in the toxicity of this mushroom it is

probably associated with other poisonous bodies which have
not yet been isolated and studied.

Muscarine is a non-protein substance with the formula
$C_5H_{15}NO_3$, which forms definite salts with acids. It is a
colourless and tasteless liquid readily miscible in water.
Another non-protein body of definite chemical composition
and possessing poisonous properties is helvellic acid, which
has been isolated from the poisonous *Helvella esculentia.*

From the highly poisonous *Amanita phalloides* toxic substances of an essentially different nature have been isolated.
Kobert in 1891 isolated a poisonous body which he considered
to be a tox-albumin and called phallin. This substance is
powerfully haemolytic. Abel and Ford (1907) consider it to
be non-protein and to be a glucoside.

Ford (1906) working with this fungus obtained two toxic
substances, one which he called amanita-haemolysin, and
identical with Kobert's phallin, and the other a-toxin.
Because of the rapidity with which it is destroyed by heat
(half-an-hour at 65° C.) and by the action of pepsin and
pancreatic juice, Ford and Bronson (1913) consider that
amanita-haemolysin is of little importance in cases of fungus
poisoning. It kills animals only slowly (three to ten days),
causing local oedema and haemoglobinuria. They regard the
a-toxin as the active poison chiefly because of its resistance
to the action of heat and the digestive ferments and because
of its ability to produce lesions in animals essentially identical
with those described for man. They do not regard it as
either a glucoside or a protein and remark that its extreme
toxicity rank it as one of the most powerful known poisons
of plant origin. These facts are in accord with the well-
known fact that these mushrooms remain after cooking intensely poisonous to man, and that while the juice of the
cooked Amanita is poisonous to animals in small doses, it is
devoid of haemolytic properties.

Poisonous parasitic growths.

The best known example of this kind of food poisoning is
the condition known as ergotism, while lathyrism is probably
a disease of this nature.

Ergotism. Practically unknown in this country and very rare now in Europe (Russia is its last home), outbreaks of ergotism or ergot poisoning were a feature of medieval Europe and epidemics seem to have been very widespread and exceedingly fatal. The condition was probably exaggerated by the bad social and sanitary condition of the peasantry especially by their chronic underfeeding. For a description of these outbreaks and a graphic account of the condition the reader is referred to the article by Allbutt in Allbutt's *System of Medicine* (2nd edition, vol. II. Part I, p. 884). Many types of symptoms were recorded and the disease ran sometimes an acute, sometimes a chronic course.

The disease was due to the consumption of rye grain affected with a vegetable parasite (*Claviceps purpurea*) forming the so-called spurred rye. *Claviceps purpurea* is a fungus attacking grain usually, but not exclusively, rye, the mycelium growth replacing the grain. The grains not displaced are discoloured and of a brownish or purple colour while the flour made from the diseased rye is correspondingly discoloured and emits a sour odour. The condition in the grain is easily recognized by microscopic examination, while there are fairly reliable chemical tests to identify it in bread and in flour.

As regards the poisonous principles of ergot up to comparatively recently the work of Kobert was followed. He found three substances: ergotine, sphacelinic acid and cornutine, and considered that they all played a part in the production of the toxic symptoms. Recent studies by Barger and Dale have demonstrated more definite toxic bodies. They have isolated two highly poisonous bodies p-hydroxyphenylethylamine and β-iminazolethylamine. Both are derived from relatively indifferent amino-acids (i.e. tyrosine and histidine respectively) by the splitting off of carbon dioxide.

Ergotism is chiefly of historical interest as a striking example of the possibility of the occurrence of widespread outbreaks of food poisoning persisting quite uncontrolled so long as the cause remained unrecognized. Even allowing for medieval exaggeration the number of victims seems to have been enormous and their sufferings appalling.

Lathyrism is another rare condition met with in certain parts of Europe (Italy, France), to a small extent in North Africa (Algeria), but especially in India.

A comprehensive contribution to the subject was made by Buchanan, I.M.S., dealing with outbreaks in India (1896–1902), while a valuable account and summary of our knowledge is given in a recent communication by Stockman (1917).

The disease occurs in man as a chronic nervous disorder due to the habitual use as a food of the peas of certain species of Lathyrus (vetchlings), the most important being *L. salivus* (S. Europe and India), *L. cicera* (France, Italy, and Algeria) and *L. clymenum* (N. Africa, the Levant and Spain). It occurs endemically and epidemically, and is first described in the writings of Hippocrates. The symptoms appear only after the peas have been eaten for some time and they vary greatly. When the peas are the sole diet the disease may appear in six to eight weeks. Individual susceptibility appears to have a considerable influence. Men are at least ten times as frequently affected as women.

The symptoms vary greatly according to the amount and period over which the peas are eaten. They usually start with cramps in the calves followed by motor paralysis of the lower limbs and often of the sphincters. A characteristic gait develops and walking is difficult and laborious. A number of other symptoms are described by different authors. Stockman points out that as very large numbers of mankind eat Lathyrus peas it is certain that when they are taken as part of a mixed dietary no poisoning results. In times of famine and poverty an excess is very apt to bring on all the symptoms of lathyrism.

Alkaloidal bodies were extracted by different workers from the peas and Stockman was able to extract a poisonous alkaloid, but only in minute quantities, which caused paralysis symptoms in monkeys.

It is possible that other grain parasites may set up food poisoning when admixed with flour. In illustration of this possibility it may be mentioned that recently (1917) a number of cases of poisoning in France have been attributed to the presence of corn-cockle (*Agrostemma githago*) in flour and bread. One sample of wheat examined by Stoecklin (1917) contained 19 per cent. of foreign seeds, including 10·2 per cent. of corn-cockle, and it is possible that contamination of wheat with this parasite is not of rare occurrence. The injurious action of corn-cockle is due to the presence of sapotoxin, and a quantity of four grms. of corn-cockle, equivalent to 0·2 grm. of sapo-toxin, produces distinctly harmful effects on adults. Sapo-toxin is best identified by means of its haemolytic action.

REFERENCES.

Animals poisonous when eaten.

Faust (1906). *Die tierischen Gifte.*
Günther (1880). *The Study of Fishes.*
Kobert (1906). *Lehrbuch der Intoxikationen.*
Mitchell (1900). *Flesh Foods.*
Miura and Takesaki (1890). *Virchow's Archiv*, CXXII. 92.
Savtschenko (1886). *Atlas der Poissons Veneneux.* St Petersburg.
Tahara (1911). *Biochemische Zeitschr.* XXX. 255.
Takahashi and Inoko (1890). *Arch. exp. Path. und Pharm.* XXVI.
    401, 453.

Poisonous plants and fungi.

Abel and Ford (1907). *Journ. Biol: Chem.*
Allbutt. *System of Medicine*, 2nd edition, Vol II. Part I. p. 884.
Cooke (1894). *Edible and Poisonous Mushrooms.* London.
Ford (1906). *Journ. Inf. Dis.* III. 191.
—— (1910). *Journ. of Pharm. and Exp. Therap.* II. 145.
—— (1910–11). *Ibid.* II. 285.
Ford and Bronson (1913). *Ibid.* IV. 241.
—— and Sherrich (1913). *Ibid.* IV. 321.
Jordan (1917). *Food Poisoning.*
McIlvaine (1912). *One Thousand American Fungi.*
Stockman (1917). *Ed. Med. Journ.* New Series, XIX. 277, 297.
Stoecklin (1917). *Analyst*, April, 1917, 142.

CHAPTER IV

FOOD IDIOSYNCRASY

THE subject of food idiosyncrasy is not of much practical importance in itself, the number of persons affected being inconsiderable. On the other hand, it is of great theoretical interest since the scientific problems which it introduces are of considerable importance. The solution of these problems may throw much light upon other types of food infection, and this possibility makes the subject of more than passing interest and indeed one worthy of detailed consideration.

It has been recognized for a long time that certain individuals are peculiarly intolerant to particular foodstuffs, the ingestion by them of such foods, even in minute quantity, being followed by a definite train of symptoms, which, however, may vary considerably in different persons. It is usual to describe such symptoms as being due to a peculiar idiosyncrasy of the individual and to dismiss the subject with this verbal subtifuge, which explains nothing. It is only in quite recent years that any scientific explanation has been forthcoming to account for this peculiarity.

Persons suffering from this food sensitiveness frequently have been affected from early infancy, while in a few cases there is a history of hereditary transmission. Lesné and Richet (1913), for example, mention a case in which idiosyncrasy to eggs existed in four generations.

The symptoms which occur usually fall into one or both of two groups, the one being disturbances of the gastrointestinal tract, shown by nausea, vomiting and diarrhoea, the other various skin affections, the commonest being urticaria, erythema and eczema. In some cases a less direct group of symptoms is met with, such as dyspnoea, incoordination of the lower limbs and attacks of asthma.

The first co-ordinating fact which emerges is that when these foods are tabulated all are found to be protein in nature

or at least to contain proteins. By far the commonest food
to cause such abnormal reactions is egg albumin, while other
foods are fish, cheese, tomatoes, buckwheat, pork and shellfish.

A few typical instances of food idiosyncrasy may be mentioned.

Galloway (1903) quotes the case of a girl who suffered
year after year from a profuse eruption of exudative erythema
with purpuric lesions. During each attack she also suffered
from entero-colitis of severe degree and haematuria lasting
for some weeks. Every autumn she was taken to the country
and as soon as she ate the first blackberries and nuts her
symptoms resulted.

Long (1913) records an extreme case of sensitiveness to
white of egg in a boy. No effect was noticed when egg was
first given to him at the age of ten months, but when next
given, when fourteen months old, after only a taste of it
"he cried out and clawed at his mouth," while his lips,
tongue and the mucous membrane of the mouth immediately
became enormously swollen, while urticarial wheals appeared
about his mouth. He did not, however, become generally
ill. Towards the end of his second year, while playing with
eggshells, urticarial wheals appeared on his hands and arms.
This occurred several times until his mother realized the cause
of the urticaria. At twenty-two months one-eighth of the
white of an egg in milk was immediately followed by swelling
of the mouth, urticaria and vomiting. Given egg-white again
when two years old more severe symptoms were present, as
not only were those mentioned above induced, but also
marked flushing, increased respiration, vomiting, muscular
twitching followed by a semi-comatose condition. Complete
recovery after three hours. In this case somewhat similar
symptoms resulted when five years old after eating an
almond and a Brazil nut.

Smith (1909) reports the case of a man who throughout
his life (first noticed when nine years old) showed a very
marked hypersensitiveness to buckwheat, the symptoms
being urticaria, angioneurotic oedema and vomiting.

McBride and Schorer (1916) collected particulars of sixty

cases of food sensitization causing skin lesions. These were more often urticaria than erythema. In their series fish, tomatoes and cheese produced only urticaria, while eggs usually were followed by urticaria, but not invariably. Cereals and pork caused erythema in a considerable percentage of the cases, the lesions usually appearing within less than four hours of eating the food; tomatoes and cereals generally produced these symptoms in less than an hour, while with fish, nuts and cheese symptoms were for the most part delayed until after four to twelve hours. The eruption itself usually lasted one to twelve hours, but in a small percentage of cases from one day to a week. In some instances there was also involvement of the respiratory tract; this varied from a slight cough to a severe dyspnoea. More than half of the cases of egg sensitization showed these symptoms, while they also occurred in a considerable proportion of those resulting from the consumption of fish, cereals and pork.

Idiosyncrasy to certain proteins may be exhibited without the absorption being of necessity through the alimentary canal, as in the extraordinary instance reported by Hollick (1903). In this case the symptoms followed the application of a hot linseed-meal poultice to an inflamed haemorrhoid. The symptoms took the form of a contracted feeling in the throat, purpuric condition of the skin with an eruption (cutis anserina), very rapid pulse, later diarrhoea and vomiting. Face and extremities cyanosed and patient in a state of collapse. These symptoms were ascribed to the linseed from the fact that on two previous occasions the man had suffered from similar, but less marked, symptoms after taking linseed. On the first occasion he had eaten a few linseed seeds, while on the second he had eaten two lozenges of linseed and liquorice.

The explanation of this interesting condition is now usually given as one of anaphylaxis. This is not a textbook of bacteriology and this complicated and difficult subject cannot be dealt with here in detail, but the following short account will explain what is meant by this hypothesis and the way this condition is supposed to arise.

It has long been recognized that the injection of protein substances, such as blood serum, into man or animals may occasionally cause poisonous symptoms, although such an injection is quite without effect in the majority of cases. It was found by Richet and others that such a condition of sensitiveness to proteins could artificially be induced in animals under certain circumstances. The easiest way such a hypersensitive condition may be set up is by the injection of a sensitizing dose of serum, insufficient in itself to produce symptoms, followed after a suitable time interval (usually about two weeks) by a second dose of serum from the same animal. This second injection, if made into a guinea-pig or other suitable animal, may be followed by very severe symptoms, with, not infrequently, collapse and death.

The minimum amount of serum necessary to bring about the symptoms of fatal anaphylactic shock is much greater, perhaps a thousand times greater, than the original sensitizing dose, while time is necessary for the anaphylactic condition to develop. The condition is specific, i.e. is manifested only on the re-injection of the same protein as that used for the sensitizing dose. Also it is to be noted that, within certain broad limits, the symptoms of anaphylactic shock are the same for each animal, no matter what the nature of the sensitizing protein employed.

If a certain quantity of the serum of an anaphylactic guinea-pig is injected into a normal guinea-pig the latter becomes anaphylactic, i.e. will give the symptoms of anaphylactic shock when serum from the animal used to sensitize is injected into it. This proves the existence of a condition of passive anaphylaxis.

Without going into questions involving the exact mechanism it may be said that the condition of anaphylaxis is one of marked hypersensitiveness to the action of foreign proteins circulating in the blood.

The matter is very well put by Wells (1918) in his *Chemical Pathology*, p. 198:

"Presumably anaphylactic intoxication is but an exaggeration of the normal process of defence of the body against foreign proteins (including bacteria) through digestion.

Normally this is accomplished in the alimentary tract and complete disintegration past the toxin stage is made certain by the presence of erepsin in the intestinal wall; but if intact foreign protein molecules reach the blood in any way, this same digestive destruction is performed by the enzymes of the blood or tissues. So abnormal is the 'parenteral' introduction of foreign proteins that, once it has happened, the protective mechanism is stimulated to the production of large amounts of proteolytic substances, and on this account if another quantity of the same protein is again parenterally introduced the breaking down of the protein is extremely rapid. Certain of the disintegration products are toxic, but with the normal rate of disintegration the amount present at any one time is inadequate to cause poisoning; when the proteolysis is accelerated as in the sensitized animal, a poisonous dose may be produced with the resulting anaphylactic intoxication. Whether this proteolysis takes place in the blood and tissues is not known."

The hypothesis that these cases of food idiosyncrasy are a variety of anaphylaxis is based on the supposition that in the individuals who exhibit the condition there is a marked hypersensitiveness to the action of particular proteins in these special foods, that they gain access to the circulation as unaltered protein and that the symptoms caused are due to individual intolerance of their presence in the blood.

There are strong arguments which suggest this as the true explanation. In the first place the symptoms induced, including the rapidity of onset (allowing time for absorption from the alimentary canal), the minute dose required, and the lesions caused, resemble in many ways those recognized as the symptoms of anaphylaxis. Further, there are many direct experiments which support this view, some of which may be mentioned.

Bruck (1909) investigated the possibility of producing experimentally a state of anaphylaxis by means of certain foods. Using hog serum and crab meat he obtained positive results with both substances in rabbits and guinea-pigs. He recorded the case of a man, aged twenty-four years, who since he was two years old could not eat pork or indeed any form of pig meat without the production of urticaria. He demonstrated that this man's serum possessed an anaphylactic antibody, and he was able to transmit this antibody to normal animals so that the injection into them of hog meat produced the typical symptoms of hypersensitiveness.

Schloss (1912) was one of the first to draw attention to the fact that the symptoms of egg idiosyncrasy in children were those of anaphylaxis. He recorded particulars of a boy of eight years who showed marked urticarial lesions following the ingestion of eggs, almonds or oatmeal. Symptoms due to eating oats appeared some time after the child had first eaten oatmeal when he was twenty-two months old. Schloss employed a cutaneous inoculation test and found this produced an urticarial wheal at the site of inoculation, this being only produced by the protein constituents of eggs, almonds or oats. He was able to immunize this patient against eggs by feeding him with ovo-mucoid (one of the active proteins in eggs) in gradually increasing doses. At the same time immunity to oatmeal and an appreciable decline in susceptibility to almonds resulted.

Schloss carried out a number of experiments to see if any protective substance was present in normal individuals but failed to find any such body. By infecting guinea-pigs intraperitoneally with some of the patient's serum it was possible to passively sensitize them to ovo-mucoid. He therefore concluded that this peculiar idiosyncrasy was due to protein sensitiveness or anaphylaxis.

Mühsam and Jacobsohn (1914) examined the sera of two patients suffering from urticaria resulting from eating crabs, and found that their sera reacted to an extract of crab albumin, so long as urticarial symptoms were present.

Bronfenbrenner, Andrews and Scott (1915) give particulars of a girl who was subject to asthmatic attacks and severe gastro-intestinal disturbances following the ingestion of small quantities of white of egg, this peculiarity having been noticed since very early childhood. By means of the Abderhalden test they demonstrated the presence of a specific antibody against the egg protein. They injected a small amount of the patient's serum into guinea-pigs thus passively sensitizing them against egg protein and subsequently repeated the Abderhalden test, using the serum of these guinea-pigs, and in this way confirmed their finding of a specific antibody against the egg protein.

The relationship of skin diseases and susceptibility to proteins has been studied by a number of workers and bears indirectly upon this question. One such investigation may be mentioned.

Blackfan (1916) used a modification of Von Pirquet's test to study the question. Superficial scarification of the skin with a needle was followed by rubbing gently the substances used into the abraded surface. A positive reaction is shown by an urticarial wheal or marked erythema and oedema at the point of scarification, appearing within a few minutes. He also used an intra-cutaneous test. His results were more particularly in relation to eczema. Of forty-three patients without eczema, only one showed any evidence of susceptibility to proteins by cutaneous and intra-cutaneous tests, while of twenty-seven patients with eczema twenty-two gave evidence of susceptibility to proteins. White of egg, cow's milk and woman's milk were the substances which most frequently caused a reaction.

Results on the same lines have been obtained by Strickler and Goldberg (1916).

Greer (1917) studied the intradermal reaction of infants suffering from gastro-intestinal disorders. He used intracutaneous injections of egg, cow's milk, and human milk albumin. Of twenty-six infants subject to gastro-intestinal disorders or atrophy resulting therefrom, twenty-three gave definite intradermal reaction with lact-albumin of the cow. Of seventeen control infants not so affected five gave a positive reaction with one or other of the substances used and three of these were cases of eczema, one gave a history of a previous severe attack of gastro-enteritis, and one of an acute and severe attack of scurvy. Greer considers that the results suggest that sensitization to cow's milk proteins does occur in acute or chronic gastro-intestinal disturbance and that lact-albumin is probably the protein to which sensitization most easily occurs.

Accepting food idiosyncrasy as being due to a condition of hypersensitization to particular proteins we have yet to consider the causes leading to the development of this condition. In a few cases the condition is hereditary but in most is acquired. Under normal conditions the intestinal mucous membrane appears to limit very sharply the passage into the circulation of any but digested protein. It has been suggested that this hypersensitive condition arises from an abnormal permeability of the intestinal mucous membrane which allows the particular protein to pass through in an unchanged state, and in this condition gain access to the blood and tissues. This foreign protein circulating in the body produces the condition of hypersensitiveness so that subsequent introductions of this protein cause the development of the symptoms of anaphylaxis.

This hypothesis is supported by the fact that Rosenau and Anderson were able in certain cases to sensitize guinea-pigs by *feeding* with horse meat and horse serum. This seems to be an inconstant phenomenon, and could not be confirmed, for example by Besredka, but is by no means improbable in view of the facts that on the one hand extremely minute doses of the protein introduced into the circulation are capable of sensitizing the body, and on the other that it has been shown that when animals are fed with proteins in large quantities they may be demonstrated as such in the circulation and even occasionally in the urine.

The interesting results of Lesné and Dreyfus (1911) bear upon this point. They injected ovo-albumin into the stomach and small intestine of rabbits and obtained no evidence of anaphylaxis, but provoked it by injections into the large intestine. It is known that substances may be absorbed from the large intestine in a comparatively unaltered condition. The earlier work of Besredka (1908, 1911), in which he found that the protection conferred upon sensitized guinea-pigs by the injection of milk into the rectum developed more rapidly and uniformly than when given by the mouth, is evidence in the same direction and suggests that the antigen is absorbed solely or chiefly from the large intestine.

Besredka (1917) in his latest monograph upon the subject

has revised some of his earlier work. He records that guinea-pigs sensitized against egg-white, milk or serum, can be made anti-anaphylactic by feeding by the mouth with these substances, but that this protection is not developed at the end of twenty-four hours, but only after the lapse of forty-eight hours or better three days. Animals so fed will resist completely an otherwise toxic dose of the sensitizing substance. Grineff has shown that (unlike its action as regards the production of anaphylaxis) heated egg-white acts in the same way as raw egg-white in conferring this immunity, suggesting that the protein is only absorbed after digestive action.

Certain of the scientific investigations which have been carried out in connection with disturbances of the infant following the introduction of artificial feeding deal with the possibility of the direct absorption of proteins from the alimentary canal, and these in general support the above contention and furnish additional data in favour of it.

Ganghofer and Langer in 1904 found that in young animals under eight days old the intestinal tract permitted the passage of heterologous proteins, such as egg or beef, using as the determining test the application of precipitin tests to the blood serum. When over eight days old this did not occur.

Somewhat similar results have been obtained by other investigators and it would appear that while the gastro-intestinal wall of the new-born infant is, or may be, permeable to foreign protein during the first few days after birth, the infant soon develops a defensive mechanism which can cope with foreign protein and prevent it reaching the blood stream in an unchanged condition. On the other hand injuries to the intestinal mucous membrane seem to be capable of breaking down these protective functions so that, in a certain proportion of such cases, foreign proteins again may pass unchanged into the blood.

Moro (1906) found that two out of twenty-two children, very ill with digestive derangements, showed the presence of foreign protein (cow casein) in the blood, as demonstrated by precipitin tests.

Lust (1913) fed infants with such foreign proteins as egg

or beef, and found (using the precipitin test applied to the urine) that they were not absorbed. On the other hand in infants suffering from acute and chronic nutritional disturbances, such as gastro-enteritis, in nine out of sixteen cases egg albumin passed unchanged through the intestinal wall, and ox serum in one out of seventeen cases.

The experiments of Hyashi (1914) were similar in their results. Schloss and Worthen (1916) have investigated the same point and come to a similar conclusion. They found the precipitin test applied to the urine for the detection of egg protein more sensitive than the anaphylactic test.

These facts suggest that the idiosyncrasy to cow's milk, which is found in certain cases, and which must be ascribed to a passage of unchanged protein through the intestinal wall, may result from sensitization during the first few days of life when the intestine is permeable, but is more likely to arise later on in infancy as a result of the passage of such proteins through an intestinal mucous membrane sufficiently damaged to allow their passage. It is also probable that the condition is favoured by a common concomitant of intestinal disturbances, an habitual excess of food.

Two good examples of idiosyncrasy to cow's milk are given by Talbot (1916).

Case 1. A healthy baby, breast fed until 8½ months old, then given one bottle of diluted cow's milk. This was taken without ill effects. No cow's milk given for three weeks; then given as whole milk and was at once vomited. A week later diluted milk was given but was vomited. Breast feeding was continued, but at the end of a further week the baby was given 1 oz. of milk with 8 ozs. of cereal gruel. Although only one teaspoonful was taken the baby shuddered when he swallowed it, vomited shortly afterwards and within an hour the body was covered with an urticarial eruption. The milk of a goat was then given and this was taken without any symptoms. Six months later cow's milk was given without further trouble.

Case 2. The mother was unable to breast feed and during the first eight weeks of life the infant was given various modifications of cow's milk, most of which were vomited.

The child had to have a wet nurse. At six different times attempts were made to wean her and she was given cow's milk in various ways, and in all sorts of modifications, but in every instance the milk was vomited and the baby became very ill. These attacks were never associated with urticaria. Scarification skin tests with fresh cow's milk, dried cow casein, the proteins of barley and potato all gave slight positive reactions. The baby was then given goat's milk, which it took without any symptoms of derangement.

REFERENCES.

Besredka (1908). *Compt. Rend. de la Soc. Biol.* LXV. 478.
—— (1911). *Ibid.* LXX. 203.
—— (1917). Monograph on *Anaphylaxie et antianaphylaxie.*
Blackfan (1916). *Am. Journ. of Diseases of Children,* XI. 441.
Bronfenbrenner, Andrews and Scott (1915). *Journ. Am. Med. Assoc.* LXIV. 1306.
Bruck (1909). *Archiv für Dermat. und Syphilis,* XCVI. 241.
Galloway (1903). *Brit. Journ. of Dermat.* XV. 235.
Greer (1917). *Archives of Pediatrics,* XXXIV. 810.
Hollick (1903). *Lancet,* II. 1428.
Hyashi (1914). *Monatschr. f. Kinderh.* XII. 749.
Lesné and Dreyfus (1911). *Compt. Rend. de la Soc. Biol.* LXX. 136.
Lesné and Richet (1913). *Archives de médecine des enfants,* XVI. 81.
Long (1913). *Journ. of Cutan. Diseases,* XXXI. 108.
Lust (1913). *Jahrb. f. Kinderh.* LXXVII. 383.
McBride and Schorer (1916). *Journ. of Cutan. and Genito-Urinary Diseases,* XXXIV. 70.
Moro (1906). *Münch. med. Woch.* LIII. 214, 2383.
Mühsam and Jacobsohn (1914). *Deut. med. Woch.* XL. 1067.
Schloss (1912). *Am. Journ. of Diseases of Children,* III. 341.
Schloss and Worthen (1916). *Am. Journ. of Diseases of Children,* XI. 342.
Smith (1909). *Arch. Int. Med.* III. 350.
Strickler and Goldberg (1916). *Journ. Am. Med. Assoc.* LXVI. 248.
Talbot (1916). *Boston Med. and Surg. Journ.* CLXXV. 409.
Wells (1918). *Chemical Pathology,* Third Edition.

CHAPTER V

THE CLINICAL AND GENERAL FEATURES OF
OUTBREAKS OF FOOD POISONING

As explained in Chapter I most food poisoning outbreaks are bacterial in origin. The present chapter is devoted to a general account of the characters of such outbreaks and a consideration of the different kinds of bacteria which have been found to be present. One group of cases, the so-called botulism, differ so materially as regards their causation, clinical features and general pathology, that they form a group apart and are most conveniently dealt with by separate presentation. This peculiar type of food poisoning is considered in Chapter IX, and the particulars given below do not apply to botulism.

The general clinical picture and other features of food poisoning outbreaks of bacterial origin are very much the same whatever the bacterial cause and although the particulars which follow are in the main based upon outbreaks due to one group of bacteria (the Gaertner group) they may be taken as generally applicable to all outbreaks of bacterial origin apart from botulism.

The following details are compiled from the analysis of a very large number (about 112) of outbreaks in this country studied by the writer, the majority of which form the basis of a comprehensive special Report to the Local Government Board (Savage, 1913) to which reference should be made for detailed particulars in regard to some special points.

The general nature of such attacks and the lines of elucidation will be best realized if a typical outbreak is described. The following one, investigated by the writer in 1908, will serve as a good illustration.

On Friday, May 8th, 1908, in Murrow, a village in Cambridgeshire a woman purchased some pork bones from a local butcher and that evening used them to make some brawn. The following morning the brawn was emptied out of the saucepan in which it had been made and, without cleansing the vessel, potatoes and asparagus were cooked in it. These vegetables were eaten for mid-day dinner by four persons and all were subsequently attacked with vomiting, diarrhoea, and the other symptoms of food poisoning, two in the night and two next morning. The husband who was away at mid-day remained well and unaffected.

On the Monday, two days later, the brawn made up into pork cheeses (a local name for brawn) was given away to three different neighbours and was consumed by a further fourteen persons, all of whom were attacked with similar symptoms, after an incubation period varying from twelve to forty-eight hours. Three of the eighteen attacked died. No one eating the brawn escaped.

None of the brawn was available for examination, but from the only fatal case investigated a Gaertner group bacillus (*B. aertrycke*) was isolated and its connection with the outbreak was further proved by the fact that it was agglutinated in high dilution by the serum of three survivors.

The brawn was home prepared and the materials were slowly heated for several hours with a short boil at the finish, but obviously actual boiling temperature was not reached. That the Gaertner bacilli were present before preparation and survived cooking is evident from the infection imparted to the vegetables through the uncleansed saucepan. Further inquiries elicited that the pig which supplied the bones for the brawn had suffered from local injury or disease of one leg, no doubt due to infection by this food poisoning bacillus.

Here are all the commonly present features of such outbreaks. A typical group of symptoms, a number of cases geographically separated but linked by a particular food consumed in common, a special bacillus demonstrated to be the pathological cause, and lastly (unlike most outbreaks) with definite evidence connecting it with disease in the animal supplying the incriminated food.

Incubation period. There is always some interval between the ingestion of the food and the onset of symptoms. The actual period varies greatly and in the writer's series of British outbreaks varied from half to forty hours or even longer. The interval most frequently recorded was from six to twelve hours. Not only does the incubation period vary in different outbreaks, but in the same outbreak widely different incubation periods have been recorded. These variations are easily explainable. In some cases the living infective bacilli are ingested with the food with none or but little of their toxic products. In such cases the incubation period will be of appreciable duration since time must elapse before the bacilli can manufacture sufficient toxins to manifest symptoms. In other cases the bacilli may be killed during the processes of manufacture, or preparation for the table, and only the heat-resisting toxic products be left. These being preformed will exert their poisonous properties rapidly. The majority of outbreaks must be looked upon as being caused by a mixture of bacilli and toxins, the bacilli having had time to grow in the food before it was consumed. In such cases varying incubation periods are likely to be met with since the amount of toxin ingested will vary with the quantity of food eaten and the degree of local bacterial contamination of the food.

Symptoms. As a rule no symptoms are present during the incubation period. The onset is usually sudden. The symptoms are essentially those of marked gastro-intestinal irritation but are frequently accompanied or followed by symptoms pointing to involvment of the nervous system.

Three symptoms—vomiting, diarrhoea and abdominal pain—are met with in almost every outbreak and frequently in every case. Vomiting is the least characteristic of these symptoms and is not invariably present. In the Chesterfield outbreak, for example, it was present in 75 per cent. of the cases.

The diarrhoea is usually very severe with repeated actions which, as a rule, are extremely offensive. Later in the attack the actions are more watery and frequently green in colour.

The abdominal pain is nearly always severe; in some outbreaks it is spoken of as agonising, and frequently is the first symptom complained of. Pain in other regions, such as the back or limbs, is not uncommon.

Prostration, marked and often persisting long into convalescence, is usually present and is a characteristic feature of most of the severe attacks. Marked collapse occurs in severe cases, often giving rise to great anxiety. Cold sweats and even rigors are mentioned as symptoms in some outbreaks.

As a rule a moderate elevation of temperature is present in the early stages of the illness. The tongue is heavily coated and the breath offensive. Headache is usually present and giddiness is frequently recorded as a symptom.

Numbness and cramp in the limbs are less commonly mentioned. Severe cramps were prominent in the Chester and also in the Wigan outbreaks.

Of other conditions which may be present the most interesting are herpes and other rashes. Herpes was recorded in a number of cases in the Bacup, Wrexham and Derby outbreaks, and rashes were specially mentioned in the Derby, Ashton-under-Lyne, Warrington and Tollesbury outbreaks. The rash is usually stated to be erythematous or urticarial in character and may be followed, as was noted in the Derby outbreak, by well-marked desquamation.

The severity of the symptoms varies very greatly in different outbreaks, and even in the same outbreak. Their duration also shows considerable variation, but symptoms usually diminish after two or three days, although marked prostration may persist much longer. Very occasionally cases with a more prostrated course are met with, the patients being ill for several weeks.

Case to case infectivity. In the records of outbreaks it is extremely rare to meet with cases of secondary infection, but a few instances are mentioned in individual outbreaks. It is probable that case to case infectivity is potentially as great as in typhoid fever, but the cases being for the most part acute and quickly ending, there is but little opportunity for secondary infection.

Age and sex distribution. There is no evidence of any

special incidence on either sex or at any age period. The age
and sex distribution in any outbreak seems to depend entirely upon the accidental age and sex distribution of those
who ate the food.

It is of interest to note that in several outbreaks instances
are recorded of babies being infected, or at least attacked
with food poisoning symptoms, through their mothers' milk,
the mothers being themselves sufferers. Thus McClure (1913)
in the Manchester outbreak mentions five such cases (ages
two weeks to fourteen months), while in the 1912 Eccles
outbreak Hamilton gives a similar case.

Infectivity rate. As a rule the infectivity rate is high. Not
infrequently all who ate the infected food became ill (100
per cent.). The *recorded* cases in individual outbreaks often
form 80 per cent. or more of those consuming the food
and is rarely under 50 per cent. Probably, however, this is
an unduly high proportion as, unless special inquiry is made
and all the food traced, attention is apt to be concentrated
upon the cases of illness and the families and individuals
overlooked who consumed the food without harm. In a
number of instances, for example, it is recorded that those
who ate the food on the day it was prepared were not
affected or were affected to a lesser extent. These cases
should all be taken into consideration when the infectivity
rate is being calculated.

Probably the form in which the food is taken, particularly
if alone or with other food, plays an important part, while
there is a certain measure of individual idiosyncrasy. For
example, in one outbreak one person ate the salmon to
which the illness was ascribed on three different occasions
and had more of it than anyone else, yet she had a comparatively mild attack, while her husband, who consumed
much less, was very ill and died.

Case mortality rate. The number of fatal cases varies
greatly in different outbreaks, as can be seen from Table I
(Addendum I). In the 112 British outbreaks mentioned in
that table, as far as the figures are available, there were
some 6190 cases with ninety-four deaths, a case mortality
rate of 1·5 per cent. For the outbreaks definitely shown to

be due to Gaertner group bacilli the case mortality rate was even lower, being 1·47 per cent.

The virulence of the particular strain of bacilli concerned, the time which it has had to grow upon the incriminated food before consumption, and the temperature of growth, are the factors which probably more especially control the mortality rate.

Pathological appearances. In severe cases the gastro-intestinal symptoms are often very intense, and it might be anticipated that very definite pathological changes would be shown in the gastro-intestinal tract in fatal cases. The changes found on post-mortem examination are, however, often slight compared with the severity of the symptoms. The mucous membrane of the stomach and intestine is swollen and congested and shows minute haemorrhagic erosions, but often nothing else. The kidneys usually show cloudy swelling, the spleen and liver are congested. These may be the only pathological appearances.

The following concisely describes the findings in a case at Wrexham, fatal after thirteen days' illness:

"The stomach was generally congested, but the congestion was more marked towards the pylorus, and several extra-vasations were noticed. The small intestines were much in-flamed, many small submucous extravasations of blood had taken place, and many patches of slight superficial ulceration were visible. The large intestine was also congested, especially the rectum. The heart was normal. The liver, kidneys and spleen were congested."

In the Limerick cases, McWeeney found that the mucous membrane of the stomach and intestines showed patches of white, prominent granules, each as large as a pin's head and consisting of nodules of tumid lymphoid tissue. The liver also showed little, indistinct pale-yellowish areas or spots, which microscopic examination showed to be due to intense fatty degeneration of the liver cells at these places. These areas are evidently similar to the necrotic areas met with in the liver, etc., of animals naturally or artificially infected with Gaertner group bacilli.

Seasonal prevalence. The influence of the time of year is

very marked, food poisoning outbreaks being far more prevalent in the hotter months. This is clearly brought out in Chart 1.

This is true of outbreaks selected without regard to etiology and applies, but not so conspicuously, when those outbreaks alone are considered, which were shown to be due to one or other member of the Gaertner group (Chart 2). It will be noticed that the months of greatest prevalence in Charts 1 and 2 are not identical, although there is a general agreement. There is not sufficient data to draw any general deduction from the differences shown.

The factor of temperature is probably insufficient in itself to explain the seasonal prevalence, and other influences may operate. It may be, for example, that Gaertner group bacilli are more virulent in the summer. The greater multiplication of these bacteria in hot weather would increase the opportunities for the transmission of infection. Flies would be more active as vehicles of infection in the summer months.

If reliable information was available as to the mean temperature at the time of each outbreak, and a sufficient number of outbreak records were available, it might be possible to draw interesting deductions between the temperature and the vehicle of infection. In Chart 3 something of the sort is attempted, the outbreaks being classified into the six groups shown and entered in the month of occurrence. No definite deductions can be drawn since the data for this purpose is vitiated by the small number of outbreaks of each group and by the fact that in any one year a spring month may be, for example, much hotter than a summer one. Assuming June, July and August as the three hot months it is of interest to note the following grouping:

Group	Total number	Number in June, July, August	Percentage in June, July, August
Made up meat foods	37	14	38
Tinned foods...	18	6	33
Fresh and not made up meat foods	20	10	50
Milk, cream and ice-cream ...	16	12	75
Viscera	5	1	20
Other foods	5	3	60
	101*	46	46

* Insufficient particulars in the other eleven cases.

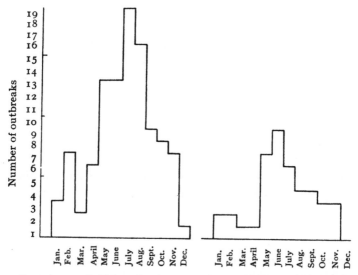

Chart 1.   112 British outbreaks.

Chart 2.   British outbreaks attributed to Gaertner group
bacilli.

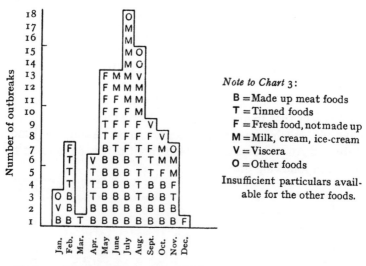

Note to Chart 3:

B = Made up meat foods
T = Tinned foods
F = Fresh food, not made up
M = Milk, cream, ice-cream
V = Viscera
O = Other foods

Insufficient particulars available for the other foods.

Chart 3.   British outbreaks with vehicle
of infection.

Physical appearance of the incriminated food. It cannot be too strongly emphasized that in the vast majority of food poisoning outbreaks the food affected is not noticeably altered in either appearance, taste or smell. The prevalent idea that the food (when some form of meat) must be, in popular parlance, "tainted" has taken a long time to become exploded and is still the prevailing view amongst the ignorant. At inquests and the like it is frequently a matter of astonishment and comment that the food found responsible for such extensive illness was not noticeably different from ordinary healthy meat.

A classical illustration is furnished by the Ghent outbreak in 1895 investigated by Van Ermengem. In this outbreak, the slaughter-house inspector (a veterinary surgeon) was so certain that the suspected meat (saveloy), in the absence of any abnormal signs, could have no connection with the outbreak that he ate two or three pieces of it, to demonstrate its harmlessness. He was attacked with severe cholera-like symptoms and died five days later, the Gaertner bacillus being recovered post-mortem.

The question of the poisonous properties of tainted meat is discussed in Chapter VII.

While no changes are noticeable in most cases to the untrained observer, in a minority of outbreaks some peculiarities such as objectionable flavour, heavy odour, moister and softer condition, etc., have been mentioned even in outbreaks definitely traced to Gaertner group bacilli. These, however, are the exception, indeed the rare exception, not the rule.

Nature of the food acting as the vehicle of infection. The great majority are spread by meat foods. In the 112 British outbreaks set out in Addendum I, in one particulars are not available as to the food or animal from which derived. In twenty-one the vehicle was a non-flesh food, i.e. milk nine, cream one, ice-cream six, potatoes two (one only probably), pineapple jelly one, canned peaches one, rice cooked in fat one. The remaining ninety were all spread by flesh foods as set out in the following table:

Table II.

Nature of the Food	Pig	Ox or Cow	Pig & Ox	Calf	Fowl	Fish	Other animals	Animal unnamed	Total
Brawn (and potted meat)	11(a)	3(b)	2	1(c)	1			1	19
Meat pies	9	3	1(d)	3				1	17
Brawn and meat pies	1								1
Meat (pork, ham, beef, etc.)	7	8	1(e)		1	4(g)	4(f)	2	27
Tinned	1	9				7(j)		2(k)	19
Sausages	1							1	2
Pickled		1							1
Internal or special organs	3(l)	1 (udder)							4
	33	25	4	4	2	11	4	7	90

(a) one with pork also.   (b) one "home pressed beef."
(c) pressed veal.   (d) with potted meat.   (e) ham and beef.
(f) rabbit, goose, shrimps and sheep (possibly), one of each.
(g) one fresh salmon, one kipper, one fried fish, one "fish."
(j) six tinned salmon, one tinned herring.   (k) both tongues.
(l) all chitterlings.

In forty-four continental outbreaks mentioned in the writer's Report to the Local Government Board, very similar findings were recorded. In three the vehicle was not meat (tinned beans two, pudding one). The others were distributed as follows:

Table III.

Nature of the Food	Pig	Ox or Cow	Pig & Ox	Calf	Fish	Horse	Sheep	Animal unnamed	Total
Flesh	4	10	1	3		2	1		21
Chopped meat	2	1				1		1	5
Sausages	3		2	1		2		2	10
Other parts	1	1		1					3
Not stated					2				2
	10	12	3	5	2	5	1	3	41

These tables show that in 68·8 per cent. of the British and 61 per cent. of the continental, where animal food was the vehicle, the animal was pig or ox. The almost complete absence of the sheep is very striking. In the one outbreak recorded in the British series which is attributed to mutton, the etiological relationship was very doubtful. In one other of these outbreaks (Surbiton, No. 23) some ribs of lamb appear to have been also secondarily affected.

When the nature of the food carrying the infection is

considered it is at once obvious what a large proportion are
due to some form of prepared meat food. Of the ninety
British outbreaks spread by meat foods, in 41 per cent.
the vehicle was brawn or meat pies, and in 21 per cent.
tinned meat or fish. Fifty-nine out of the whole, or almost
exactly two-thirds, were spread by such prepared foods, while
three further cases were due to chitterlings. When the
twenty-seven remaining cases are considered in detail it is
found that in a good many of these the food was not simply
the freshly cooked meat. They include several instances in
which the meat was stuffed before roasting, in others it was
twice cooked and was only harmful after standing and being
warmed up next day, in others the meat was ham or other
forms which are really prepared foods. In a good number
the particulars recorded are very indefinite and inadequate.
When allowance is made for this and the other points mentioned it is evident that the number of cases in which the
meat food was not subjected to some special form of preparation other than simple cooking is a very small proportion of
the whole.

Apart from tinned fish the number of cases ascribed to
fish is small, and in view of the considerable possibilities of
contamination smaller than might be expected. A number
of continental outbreaks have however been described, for
example, Ulrich (1906, several kinds of fish), Abraham (1906,
pike), Reinhold (1912, halibut) and Müller (1914, fried eels).

The incidence on milk and its relation to disease of the cow
is dealt with on page 161.

Bacteria detected in food poisoning outbreaks. In the British
outbreaks analysed and set out in the table (Addendum I)
it will be noted that Gaertner group bacilli were isolated in
a large number of cases. Excluding outbreaks reported
before 1890, when bacteriological technique was not well
advanced, and thirty-five outbreaks in which no bacteriological examinations at all were made, the results in the remaining sixty-two outbreaks were as follows:

```
Gaertner group bacilli detected      ...    ...    ...    ...   =43
No Gaertner bacilli found:
    Very incomplete bacteriological examination...    ...   = 9
    More extensive    ...    ...    ...    ...    ...    ...   =10
```

The nine outbreaks with very incomplete bacteriological examination hardly merit further consideration as the examinations made were, in most cases, most inadequate, and Gaertner group bacilli if present would readily be missed.

In the majority of the ten outbreaks in which a fairly complete bacteriological examination was made but no Gaertner group bacilli were isolated, no examinations were made from any of the patients, but were confined to an investigation of the supposed peccant material. For several of these there was some doubt as to whether the food submitted for examination was the same as that which caused the illness. For example, in the Cambridge (1914) outbreak due to fresh salmon, three fish were cooked weighing sixty pounds and although the salmon left over after the feast was submitted for examination it may well have been derived from a non-infected fish since only 95 out of 196 (48 per cent.) who consumed the salmon were attacked. No specimens from sufferers were examined. In another of these ten outbreaks (No. 60) the steak and kidney pie examined by the writer was one of a batch of four, of which two only had been eaten with harmful results, and since no part of the pie examined had been consumed it may possibly have been free from the bacilli which were evidently present in the other two. In several of the cases no agglutination reactions with the blood of the patients were carried out.

In one of these outbreaks (Westminster, No. 99) agglutination tests were carried out and three out of six sera specimens from patients agglutinated Gaertner group bacilli, so that this outbreak was probably due to Gaertner toxins, the negative results in the other cases being due to smallness of the dose of toxins. This outbreak is not included as due to this group as there is this element of doubt.

In outbreak No. 107 (Glasgow) the bacteriological examination was negative and the outbreak was ascribed to solanine (see page 145).

In but few of these outbreaks was a complete examination made. It is further noteworthy that in only one of these ten outbreaks was there a fatal case (No. 99) and this was the one, as mentioned above, which was probably due to

Gaertner infection, while no bacteriological examinations at all were made of the organs of the fatal case. Out of thirty in the series of ninety-seven outbreaks since 1890 in which deaths resulted and in which a bacteriological examination was made, in twenty-eight Gaertner group bacilli were detected. In one case the bacteriological examination was negative, the outbreak being ascribed to solanine, while the remaining case was the Westminster outbreak, which was probably a Gaertner infection.

While this may be advanced by some as showing that the less severe outbreaks are not always due to Gaertner group bacilli it should be remembered that the true bacterial cause of any outbreak of food poisoning is far more likely to be ascertained if the organs of fatal cases are available for examination. The failure to find Gaertner bacilli in cases in which there were no deaths may, in at least many outbreaks, be ascribed to the unsatisfactory nature of the material available for examination. The bacteriological examination of the incriminated food itself may be difficult and unsatisfactory, in part due to delay in transmission to the bacteriologist, in part to the growth of other organisms which may obscure or even totally eliminate the bacillus reponsible for the outbreak, and in part to the possibility that the food submitted for examination is either not part of that incriminated or that the particular portion selected for examination is free from the bacilli concerned in the outbreak.

In no instance was it possible to advance proof that any other bacillus was the cause of the outbreak of food poisoning.

While therefore out of the sixty-two outbreaks in which a bacteriological examination was made Gaertner group bacilli were only detected forty-three times (70 per cent.), in but few of the remaining attacks was a complete and satisfactory examination made, and it cannot be doubted that the percentage would be much higher if more thorough and extensive investigations had been done.

In every one of the forty-one continental outbreaks set out in Table III one or other member of the Gaertner group of bacilli was isolated.

These figures suggest that outbreaks of food poisoning and

food infections are in the main due to the activities of one
or another member of the Gaertner group and that the share
of other bacilli is negligible, at least as regards definite widespread outbreaks. As regards the indefinite attacks of illness
with food poisoning symptoms, usually limited to one or two
families or even to one or two individuals, which follow the
consumption of certain articles of food, our knowledge as to
causation is very inadequate since so few are fully investigated. Since when they are examined a considerable proportion is found to be due to Gaertner group bacilli we are
justified in assuming that at least many of these have an
etiology similar to the more definite outbreaks.

From the point of view of causation we can divide food
poisoning outbreaks of bacterial origin into three groups:

(a) Those due to Gaertner group bacilli—the great majority
of the large outbreaks.

(b) Cases of botulism. An insignificant group due to *B.
botulinus*.

(c) Those due to the toxic action of bacteria other than
the above.

Of the third group the most important place is usually
ascribed to putrefactive bacteria such as *B. coli* and *B.
proteus*. The characters of the Gaertner group are considered
in Chapter VI, botulism in Chapter IX, and the relationship
of putrefactive bacteria to food poisoning in Chapter VII.
In the present chapter there only remains to be considered
the evidence incriminating other bacteria as a cause of food
poisoning.

Apart from its activities as a putrefactive bacillus some
suspicion and many unfounded assertions have gathered
round *B. coli* as a cause of food poisoning. Inasmuch as the
B. coli group (using the expression in a comprehensive sense
to include *B. coli communis* and a number of allied forms)
comprises organisms of very varying virulence, some of
which may be decidedly pathogenic to man, it is a quite
possible supposition.

On the other hand in none of the extensive series of outbreaks in this country which the writer has studied could
any member of this group of organisms be claimed as the

cause. They were frequently present in the foodstuffs examined but no etiological connection was established. Their
being present is of no significance since they are usually
present in large numbers in identical but non-poisonous foodstuffs (ice-cream, brawn, etc.).

In some of the earlier continental outbreaks, for example,
Grünthal (1895) and Glückstadt (1896), *B. coli* is ascribed
as the cause, but as Fischer (1902) points out, and as is obvious
from the records, the proof is most incomplete. The association of this organism with unfit cheese is better substantiated
(see p. 138).

Other bacilli have been suggested in individual outbreaks.

Parkes (1905) describes an interesting series of cases of
diarrhoea which continually occurred amongst the inmates
of a large country mansion. The larder had recently been
altered, and since then the meat and some other foods kept
in the larder showed a pink growth. This was examined and
identified as *B. prodigiosus*. The larder was cleaned out
and disinfected and subsequently there was no diarrhoea or
B. prodigiosus growth. As Parkes himself is careful to point
out the chain of evidence is incomplete and is only suggestive.

B. prodigiosus is not, in general, a pathogenic organism,
and indeed has been used extensively to inoculate the human
mouth in experiments, and this without any harm. On the
other hand Woodward and Clarke (*Lancet*, 1913, CLXXXIV.
314) describe a case in which this bacillus was found as
the probable cause of chronic cough and offensive sputum.

Rappin (1913) under the name *B. hypertoxicus* describes
an organism to which he ascribes an outbreak of food
poisoning affecting twenty persons, with one death, the
vehicle being clotted cream and milk. The characters given
in the paper are indefinite, but it was lactose positive and
probably a variety of *B. coli*. A study of the paper shows
that the evidence that the organism had anything to do
with the outbreak is of the weakest, but the outbreak is
mentioned here since Rappin also states that he has isolated
this bacillus from other cases in the course of an epidemic of
similar illness in another place. *B. faecalis alkaligenes* has
now been established as a cause of illness of the type of

typhoid fever under certain conditions[1], while Ridder (1909) has shown it to be the probable cause of a single sporadic case of gastro-enteritis following the consumption of some pickled and smoked pork, but the writer has been unable to find any evidence connecting it with an outbreak of food poisoning.

While therefore there is a likelihood, or at least a possibility, that individual cases and even widespread outbreaks may be due to *B. coli* or bacilli other than those of the Gaertner group, there is no clear evidence connecting them with any definite outbreaks, and records of such cases require to be very clearly demonstrated before they can be accepted.

REFERENCES.

To save repetition the References for Chapters V, VI and X are given together at the end of Chapter X.

[1] For example see Rochaix and Marotte, 1916, *Compt. rend. de la Soc. de Biologie*, LXXIX. 316, and Shearman and Moorhead, 1916, *Brit. Med. Journ.* II. 893.

CHAPTER VI

THE GAERTNER, OR SALMONELLA, GROUP OF BACTERIA (IN RELATION TO FOOD POISONING)

THE colon-typhoid group of bacteria is one of great size and complexity and may be classified in various ways. Contained in it and intermediate between *B. typhosus* at one end and the *B. coli* family at the other is the important and fairly distinctive series of organisms, the Gaertner (or Salmonella) group or, as it is frequently called, the Paratyphoid-Enteritidis group.

The following characteristics are common to all members of the Gaertner group: short, sporeless bacilli, with rounded ends, motile and usually markedly motile, gram negative; grow on gelatine as a white or translucent growth without liquefaction; produce at first some acid in litmus milk then after a few days incubation at 37° C. (the exact time may vary with different strains) marked alkali production; milk is never clotted; do not produce indol; glucose and mannite are fermented with the production of acid and gas, while lactose and saccharose are not fermented, neither acid nor gas being produced.

B. paratyphosus A does not produce alkalinity in milk when the incubation period is not prolonged but is usually considered a member of the group. As regards this point a number of observers (for example, Bradley (1912), Krumwiede, Pratt and Kohn (1916 *b*) and Jordan (1917)) have recently shown that this difference in milk between the Paratyphoid *A* and *B* strains is one of degree only and that, given a sufficient period of observation, many if not all *A* strains will produce alkalinity in milk.

Jordan, for instance, found that twenty *A* strains all remained more acid than the control tube for nearly two weeks, but in about fourteen to fifteen days at 37° C. many approximated to the reaction of the control and then became progressively alkaline. After about five weeks the alkalinity was distinct but even then was considerably less than for B strains.

Jordan (1918 b) in a later paper has further studied this point. He obtained the interesting result that the A strains multiply much less rapidly than the B strains in milk and considers that the differences between the A and B types in rapidity of alkali formation in milk is largely, if not altogether, a numerical relation due to gradations in the amount and rate of multiplication.

On the other hand investigators have recently advanced another cultural test to distinguish the A and B types. Krumwiede, Pratt and Kohn (1916 a), confirming an earlier observation of Ford (1905), found that all B. *paratyphosus A* strains failed to ferment xylose, unlike the *enteritidis-paratyphoid B* strains. Weiss obtained the same results and so has Jordan.

Some authors describe the production of indol by these bacilli, but a large number of strains from many different sources tested by the writer always yielded negative results, which is in accord with the work of Jordan and many other workers.

The group can be sub-divided into two sub-groups:

A. True Gaertner bacilli.

B. Para-Gaertner bacilli.

The true Gaertner bacilli are for the most part culturally indistinguishable and in addition to the above characters they ferment dulcite, maltose, galactose, laevulose, and xylose, while they do not ferment salicin, raffinose or glycerine. In glycerine they may produce a little acid, but never gas.

The writer has given the name of para-Gaertner bacilli to a number of organisms, for the most part unnamed, which appear to be not uncommon in the healthy animal and human intestine, and which are of interest on account of their close resemblance to the true pathogenic members. He first drew attention to their presence in a series of Reports to the Local Government Board (1906–7, 1907–8, 1908–9), finding them in quite small numbers in the human intestine but rather more abundant in the healthy animal intestine.

They can be distinguished culturally by an extended series of fermentation tests, especially of dulcite and salicin. They frequently fail to ferment dulcite while fermenting salicin, the exact opposite of the true strains. That these differences are real and distinctive is shown by the fact that these strains fail to be agglutinated by the sera of animals immunized by the different types of true Gaertner bacilli, while the sera of animals injected with repeated doses of these para-Gaertner strains do not agglutinate the true types. They are non-pathogenic and do not produce heat-resisting toxins.

The true Gaertner strains can be further sub-divided by means of serological tests. The strains so far isolated, with a few unimportant exceptions, can be divided into three types, but others may become known. These are:

(a) B. enteritidis. Includes not only many of the Gaertner bacilli isolated from food poisoning outbreaks but also several of the rat viruses (such as Danysz bacillus) and some strains of B. typhi murium. Agglutination tests easily differentiate this bacillus from the other types.

(b) B. paratyphosus B. The organism causing paratyphoid fever of the B type and also found in the human intestine in carrier cases.

(c) B. suipestifer. Includes a number of the food poisoning bacilli, some B. typhi murium strains and probably B. psittacosis. The strains isolated from cases of swine fever (hog cholera) belong to this group. Many strains from these cases have been labelled B. suipestifer while showing distinct cultural differences and some confusion has resulted. It should only be applied to bacteria with the above cultural characters.

In nearly all German literature the B. suipestifer and B. paratyphosus B sub-groups are considered to be identical and only two sub-types are recognized. By agglutination and especially by absorption tests it is, however, possible to distinguish definitely between these two strains (Bainbridge, Savage, etc.). This view has recently been confirmed by the extended cultural, agglutination and absorption tests of Krumwiede, Kohn and Valentine (1918).

As mentioned above all these strains are usually considered to be culturally identical, but Jordan (1917) in a recent valuable comparative study of strains of Gaertner group organisms from different sources found cultural differences in the strains isolated from diseased swine fever pigs. These *B. suipestifer* organisms in his hands attacked arabinose and dulcite slowly or not at all, both substances being fermented rapidly by the other sub-groups. Jordan and Victorson (1917) found that the same *B. suipestifer* strains failed to blacken lead acetate paper, a characteristic quality of all the *B. enteritidis* and *B. paratyphosus B* organisms. Weiss (1916) also records variations as regards the fermentation of inosite.

Trawinski (1918) studied forty-two *B. suipestifer* strains from an epidemic of swine fever occurring at a pig-depot for swine from Poland. The strains isolated all differed culturally from *B. paratyphosus B* only in the fact that they failed to ferment dulcite and arabinose and produced acid but no gas in sorbite.

All these strains were isolated from pigs and were therefore of direct animal origin, and these cultural differences do not appear to occur with the strains isolated from food poisoning outbreaks, and which on cultural and serological tests are called *B. suipestifer* as they can be distinguished from *B. paratyphosus B*. If these conclusions as to cultural differences are confirmed it may be necessary to sub-divide the true Gaertner strains into four instead of three sub-groups, i.e. *B. enteritidis*, *B. paratyphosus B*, *B. aertrycke* and *B. suipestifer*, the *B. suipestifer* group mentioned on page 63 being divided into true *B. suipestifer* strains with the cultural differences shown by Jordan and of purely porcine origin, and *B. aertrycke* strains, those culturally identical with *B. paratyphosus B* but of human origin and distinguishable by agglutination and absorption tests.

A further point in connection with the cultural characters of this group is the possibility of variation of cultural and biological characters.

Penfold (1911) has drawn attention to the possibility of obtaining considerable variability in the gas-forming powers of intestinal bacteria and by using special means obtained a

diminution of the gas-producing power of *B. enteritidis.*
These methods, however, were more or less artificial and
can hardly compare with those produced under more or less
natural conditions.

Ten Broeck (1916) records particulars of a hog-cholera
strain (*B. suipestifer*) which after passage through a series
of rabbits produced acid, but failed to form gas, from dulcite,
mannite, maltose, glucose, galactose and laevulose, a feature
which persisted over a' period of eighteen months in spite of
varied attempts to induce the strain to revert to its original
characters. In pathogenic and agglutination properties it
was unaltered from the original.

Dorset, Moore, Bock and others have recorded strains of
B. suipestifer which failed to ferment glucose with gas production.

The writer (Savage and Forbes, 1918) in an extensive food
poisoning outbreak due to fried fish isolated a strain which
on its other characters was identical with *B. enteritidis*, but
which when isolated, both from the fatal case and from the
human carrier causing the outbreak, failed to produce gas
in mannite and dulcite, and only produced a single bubble
of gas in glucose; acid was however produced. Passage
through a guinea-pig failed to alter these abnormalities.
After artificial cultivation in litmus milk and other media
for several weeks moderate gas production with glucose
and dulcite and well-marked gas production in mannite
was obtained.

While therefore the cultural characters of this group are
in general very definite and well marked there may occasionally be met with some abnormalities as regards fermentation
properties, chiefly or entirely in the direction of a temporary
suppression or retardation.

Hutchens and Tulloch (1914) isolated an organism from
yeast from a brewery culturally identical with *B. paratyphosus B* which showed anomalous agglutination and absorption reactions. While, in general, these tests are definite,
anomalies are occasionally met with.

Gaertner group bacilli as disease-producing organisms.

These organisms are etiologically associated with a number of diseases and as this relationship is of very great importance in connection with the causation of food poisoning, detailed consideration of the subject is necessary.

Disease in man. Apart from certain exceptional cases these organisms have been found associated with only two conditions, viz., cases of paratyphoid fever and outbreaks of food poisoning.

It is only comparatively recently that paratyphoid fever has been separated from enteric fever (for example, two cases described by the writer in 1905 were amongst the earliest recorded cases in this country), but it is now well recognized as a separate disease. The clinical features are nearly indistinguishable from enteric fever, being chiefly characterised by a lessened severity, and to distinguish the two diseases bacteriological tests are necessary. Like enteric fever there is no evidence that this disease affects the lower animals. A proportion of the cases are due to *B. paratyphosus A*, but the majority (at least in Europe) are due to *B. paratyphosus B*.

There are very few instances in which *B. enteritidis* has been found to cause human disease, apart from food poisoning outbreaks. Two in this country may be mentioned.

Batten and Forbes (1908) describe two cases of infection of infants with *B. enteritidis*. They suffered from diarrhoea and vomiting with considerable fever, the symptoms persisting for a number of weeks and ending fatally in both instances. The two cases were quite unconnected and no evidence was available as to how they became infected. Both had been fed upon cow's milk and the bacilli may have gained access from this source.

Dean (1911) has described a case of suppurative cholecystitis with cholelithiasis in a woman of sixty-one years. *B. enteritidis* was isolated from the pus, gall bladder and stools. There was no history of acute food poisoning. The serum of the patient agglutinated the bacillus in low dilution. The case is of interest as the bacilli were excreted intermittently in the excreta in the same way as in typhoid and paratyphoid fever carriers.

Disease in animals. In animals members of the Gaertner group appear to play a considerable disease-producing rôle and in this way are sharply separated from the allied typhoid bacillus which is incapable, so far as is known, of producing a natural disease in animals. The writer has been at some labour to investigate the literature, in view of its importance in relation to food poisoning, but in order not to obscure the balanced presentation of the subject the details are relegated to an Addendum (No. II) to this chapter, only a general account being given here.

In swine fever organisms of this group (*B. suipestifer*) have been found in a variable proportion of cases, the actual percentages ranging from 0 to 50 or over, not as the cause of the disease, but associated with the filterable virus generally accepted as the primary cause. An accurate bacteriological classification has not always been adhered to and in some cases the organisms found cannot be accepted as members of the group.

Members of this group of bacilli have also been isolated from calves associated with a number of diseased conditions, especially septicaemia and calf dysentery.

As long ago as 1876 Bollinger recognized the frequent association of outbreaks of food poisoning in man with the consumption of the meat of animals suffering from pyaemic and septicaemic conditions, and Gaertner group bacilli have been isolated from cows suffering from udder inflammation and occasionally from septic conditions or enteritis in the domestic animals generally.

In horses they have been found by several observers associated with outbreaks of abortion in mares, although they are not the common cause of this condition.

In a good many instances they have caused epidemics of disease in birds, such as parrots, canaries, pigeons and finches.

They are a not uncommon cause of disease in rats and mice, and to a lesser extent amongst other small rodents, causing widespread epidemics.

While it is clear from the above summary that the Gaertner group of bacilli are responsible for a considerable amount of disease in animals as in man, a careful study of the individual outbreaks makes it evident that while they do play a disease-producing rôle in animals they are not the most common or even the most usual cause of the pathological condition with which they are associated. They occur as infrequent causes of the condition while in many cases they may only exert a secondary disease-producing effect. This important point will be considered further when the causation of food poisoning outbreaks is dealt with in Chapter X.

Distribution of Gaertner group bacilli in nature apart from pathological conditions.

Not a little of the existing deficiencies in our knowledge as to the exact causes and sources of infection in food poisoning outbreaks are due to the conception, largely based in the writer's view on conclusions from faulty observations in Germany, that this group of bacilli are natural intestinal inhabitants of the domestic animals and even of man. The writer started his investigations upon the causation of food poisoning in 1905 with this as a possible hypothesis and starting point, but detailed searching investigations soon convinced him of its inaccuracy, while the detection of the para-Gaertner bacilli furnished a feasible explanation of where these continental workers had gone astray, as for the most part these organisms would be included by them as true Gaertner group bacilli.

This question is of such great significance in connection with the sources of infection in food poisoning outbreaks, while some of the results have been so discrepant, that it is necessary to discuss it in considerable detail. To avoid overloading the text proper with details, the results of the different investigations are set out in a separate Addendum (No. III), leaving to be included here a general summary of the facts obtained. The available data as to distribution may be conveniently grouped as follows: in the human intestine, in the animal intestine, in fresh and prepared meat.

(a) *In the human intestine.* While a few of the earlier German investigators record the presence of Gaertner group bacilli in the excreta of healthy persons, the majority of recent German workers have failed to find these bacilli apart from actual cases of disease, or persons acting as carriers after infection. All English investigators have been unable to find these bacilli in the contents of healthy human excreta, except in extremely rare instances.

The available data justifies the conclusion that *B. paratyphosus B* and other members of the group are not present in the normal healthy human intestine, or even in pathological conditions, unless the disease is paratyphoid fever or other condition in which these bacilli play a disease-producing rôle. When therefore they are found they suggest either the existence of a Gaertner caused disease or that the person is acting as a carrier of these bacilli after infection.

(b) *In the animal intestine.* An extended series of investigations has been carried out. The earlier continental workers claimed to have found these bacilli in considerable numbers in the intestine of quite healthy food producing animals and founded upon their work it became widely accepted that these bacilli were normal inhabitants of the animal intestine, at least of some animals. The writer and others, however, demonstrated that this view could not be maintained and that the claim of the ubiquitous presence of these organisms in the animal gut was probably due to an insufficient series of differentiating tests being carried out, and that when proper steps were taken to exclude these para-Gaertner forms, genuine Gaertner bacilli were not found. Later continental investigations with better technique have failed to find these bacilli in any numbers and the balance of evidence may be said to show conclusively that these bacilli are not *natural* inhabitants of the animals used for food and that they are not found more frequently than can be accounted for on the supposition that their presence is due to an actual case of disease or the carrier state after infection.

In view of the extensive contamination of food by rats and mice considerable interest centres in the question as to how far members of this group of organisms are present in these animals and some writers have suggested that they may be the natural reservoir for these bacilli. Here again, however, investigations lead to the conclusion that these organisms are not natural inhabitants and do not occur in a higher percentage than can be accounted for on the supposition of a carrier state in a class of animals which are very susceptible to infection from members of this group.

(c) *In meat, particularly prepared meat.* A large number of samples of such foods have been examined and the results show that while members of this group of bacilli are nearly always absent they are very occasionally found to be present, probably due to contamination from an animal case or carrier, or in rare instances from a human carrier. Such meat must be regarded as a potential source of disease.

The general result of all these investigations, as the writer construes them, is that the Gaertner group of bacilli are important causes of disease in both man and the lower animals, but that these organisms are not found under healthy normal conditions. For example, they cannot like *B. coli*, or some of the allied non-lactose fermenting strains, be accepted as normal inhabitants of the intestine, but like *B. typhosus* they only occur either associated with definite disease or in the carrier state, as the result of persistence after the pathological condition has subsided or after a definite infection, which, however, may have been too slight to have set up recognizable objective symptoms.

Special characters of the Gaertner group in relation to food poisoning.

There are several properties possessed by this group of bacilli which are probably of considerable practical importance and which throw a good deal of light upon a number of perplexing points in connection with the methods of infection by the group.

(a) *Variable pathogenicity.* When first isolated from the animal body these bacilli usually possess considerable pathogenicity towards the lower animals, especially when inoculation methods are employed. This applies to all three varieties and no essential differences are observable between

the different members. Most observers are agreed that
virulence is rather rapidly lost when the bacilli are kept
under artificial conditions, although considerable variability
is shown with different strains. There is some discrepancy
of evidence as to how far the virulence of such strains can
be restored by special cultural methods or by animal passage.
Gaertner noted that while the infective power of the bacillus
may not be greatly impaired, the organism rather rapidly
loses its power of producing toxins, an observation confirmed
by later observers. Holst found, using the bacillus isolated
by him from the Gaustad Asylum outbreak, that the toxin-
producing capacity, after rapidly diminishing, could be
restored by several passages of the bacillus through pigeons.
Van Ermengem found that the bacillus isolated by him from
the Moorseele outbreak (*B. enteritidis*) behaved in the same
way. Rolly found that the Gaertner organism isolated by him in
connection with an outbreak from tinned beans was harmless
to mice by feeding but caused death in 4–7 days after passage
through three mice. Trautmann obtained an increase of
virulence by growth upon sterilized meat or upon pigeon
blood agar and a diminution when grown upon ordinary
agar, while he obtained decrease of virulence by animal
passage. Xylander (1908*a*) found an increase followed by a
decrease by animal passage. Kosche (1906) found an increase
by intracranial rabbit passage. Heuser, using bacilli of the
hog-cholera group, found distinct increase of virulence by
animal passage through rats, but did not obtain a bacillus
capable of causing infection by feeding. Smith and Reagh
(1903) passed a hog-cholera strain through a series of fourteen
rabbits and increased its virulence 10,000-fold (from 0·1 c.c.).
Ten Broeck passed another hog-cholera strain through
eleven rabbits and increased its virulence a thousand times
for subcutaneous inoculation, but unfortunately no feeding
experiments were recorded.

The strains which have been employed for exterminating
rats and mice (see p. 176) differ in no cultural or agglutination
qualities from true Gaertner group bacilli, and are now considered to be identical with them except that they show, for
the most part, low pathogenicity to human beings. To this

fact must be ascribed the comparatively few cases of human infection, compared with the abundant opportunities afforded. Whether, on the other hand, these bacilli can acquire markedly increased virulence for man and so be capable of originating definite disease symptoms is an important point upon which we possess very little evidence.

Another point of considerable significance is the great variability met with when the method of infection is by feeding. Evidence of infection of animals by feeding is mentioned in connection with a number of outbreaks of which the following may be mentioned as examples. The bacilli isolated from the outbreaks at Wrexham, St Annes-on-the-Sea, and Accrington when used to feed mice or guinea-pigs caused infection and death. In the Partick outbreak in one house the cat ate a good deal of the infected meat. The animal suffered from extreme sickness, vomiting and purging, and continued after the subsidence of the acute symptoms in a lethargic state for several days. In connection with the Tollesbury outbreak a dog ate some of the infected brawn and was taken ill, but recovered.

Pottevin (1905) carried out a careful experiment with a cat, feeding it with milk in which a bacillus, which had caused a food poisoning outbreak, had been grown for forty-eight hours. The cat became ill and suffered from diarrhoea for three weeks then gradually recovered. The bacillus was isolated from the excreta for over a month while the serum of the cat at the end of the illness developed well-marked powers of agglutination against this bacillus.

On the other hand the bacilli isolated by the writer from the Murrow outbreak and by McWeeney from the Limerick outbreak, although both virulent to laboratory animals by injection, did not cause infection by feeding, and the same fact is recorded in other outbreaks.

Kutscher and Meinicke (1906) carried out a large series of feeding experiments, with, in general, negative results. Negative results were obtained with rats, rabbits, dogs and goats fed with B. paratyphosus B. Two sheep fed with the same bacillus showed a rise of temperature but no other definite symptoms. Ten guinea-pigs fed did not show any symptoms but developed an active immunity against this bacillus. Feeding experiments with white and grey mice were usually negative but two particular strains constantly killed white mice in from eight to fourteen days. It was not found possible to raise the virulence for feeding by animal passage. Two 2–3 weeks old calves were made violently ill with diarrhoea, temperature elevation, etc., but completely recovered, while they did not develop agglutination properties nor could the bacilli be recovered from the foetid slimy stools.

Reinhardt and Seibold (1912 a) fed a goat with a strain of B. enteritidis which was very virulent to goats when injected intraperitoneally into the udder or knee joint, and which previously had been passed through four goats. Some slight rise of temperature was noted but there was no noticeable effect upon the health of the animals and when killed there were no lesions, while the organs were sterile. The dose given was the whole of an agar culture every day for five days.

The same authors give an interesting instance of a case of natural infection which throws light upon the way these diseases may be spread. A goat was infected by the injection of an emulsion of four agar cultures into the uterus, this causing marked illness. The three kids of this goat born two days before the inoculation were removed from their mother but were brought back in the evenings and drank her milk. Two remained unaffected but the third sickened eight days after the mother was infected and died three days later, showing gastritis and duodenal catarrh *post mortem*. The bacillus was readily isolated from the internal organs.

A very interesting instance of human infection apart from a food poisoning outbreak is recorded by Meyer (1916). A man aged twenty-six years was infected in connection with the feeding of a calf with sterilized milk containing a B. enteritidis strain, isolated from a calf naturally infected with this bacillus. After an incubation period of ten to twelve hours he was attacked with severe abdominal cramps, nausea, severe diarrhoea, flatulence, headache and some rise of temperature. The symptoms persisted for several days, but he recovered completely within a week. The bacillus was readily isolated from his excreta while he developed agglutinins against this organism. Several other men ran an equal risk of being infected and Meyer considers that the important predisposing factor was that this man had been and was at the time of infection suffering from a chronic mucous colitis.

These variable feeding results are recorded in some detail since we are dealing with a disease which invariably is acquired by way of the mouth, and which exerts its effects mainly upon the alimentary tract. It may be that the vehicle of infection is of importance and that infection is more likely to result when introduced upon foodstuffs than when the naked bacilli are given, also whether or no the bacilli are introduced with their specific toxins may affect the likelihood of actual infection resulting.

(b) *Nature of the toxins.* A further point of importance is the nature of the toxins produced by these bacilli. The experimental data is discrepant as to whether these bacilli join the very small band of organisms which produce true toxins (extra-cellular) or whether the toxins are contained in the bodies of the bacilli (endo-toxins). Cathcart, for example, as well as a number of other workers, such as Brion and Kayser, Kutscher and Meinicke, Levy and Fornet, found no evidence of soluble toxins, while others such as Uhlenhuth, Zwick and Weichel found evidence of toxic bodies in filtrates. One of the most recent investigations is by Ecker (1917), which may be consulted for a review of the literature, who, working with *B. paratyphosus B*, concluded that in broth cultures soluble toxic substances are produced within twenty-four hours by some strains of this organism. He found that these toxic substances produced constant pathological effects and that they were of the nature of true soluble toxins, inasmuch as they stimulate the formation of antitoxins. The toxic substances are comparatively thermostable since they resist boiling for five minutes at 100° C.

(c) *Heat resistance.* A further point of great interest is the resistance of members of this group to heat. They all behave alike, and being non-sporing bacilli are fairly easily killed, a comparatively short exposure (thirty minutes) at 60° C.

being sufficient to ensure their destruction. Their toxins, on the other hand, are characteristically heat-resistant. This was first shown by Gaertner with the original *B. enteritidis* isolated by him, and has since been confirmed by very numerous investigators. Van Ermengem, for example, found the toxins of his Moorseele bacillus (*B. enteritidis*) to resist heating to 100° C. or even up to 120° C. Cathcart found that both *B. enteritidis* and *B. paratyphosus B* toxins withstood heating to 100° C. for thirty minutes.

As shown by Gaertner, Fischer, Holst and others, the production of heat-resisting toxins is a property which rapidly becomes lost when the bacilli are artificially cultivated outside the animal body.

This remarkable power of resistance to heat possessed by the toxins of this group explains the fairly numerous outbreaks which are due to food materials which contain no living Gaertner group bacilli. The bacilli are killed during the process of preparation for sale, but the pre-formed toxins persist in virtue of their heat-resisting properties.

ADDENDUM I.

TABLE I. BRITISH OUTBREAKS.

Number	Place	Year	Month	Incubation period (in hours)	Number of Cases	Deaths	Kind of food eaten	Animal from which derived	Bacteria isolated
1	Whitchurch	1878	—	4–19	—	2	Roast leg of pork	Pig	—
2	Welbeck	1880	June	12–36 for most	72 +	4	Cold ham	Pig	The Welbeck bacillus.
3	Nottingham	1881	February	7–24	15	1	Hot baked pork	Pig	No bacteria isolated.
4	Oldham	1882	—	½–5	9	0	Tinned tongues	Pig	
5	Bishop Stortford	1882	—	—	3 families	0	Ribs of beef	Ox	—
6	Whitchurch	1882	May	1–5	10 families	0	Brawn	Pig	—
7	Wolverhampton	1884	—	10–14	3	2	Tinned salmon	Salmon	—
8	Carlisle	1886	August	6–43	20	1	—	—	—
9	Iron Bridge	—	—	6–12	12	0	Veal pies	Calf	—
10	Retford	1887	November	6–30	80	1	Pork pies and brawn	Pig	—
11	Carlisle	1889	November	about 24	25	0	Pork pies and boiled salt pork	Pig	A bacillus.
12	Portsmouth	1890	February	14–17	12	0	Meat pies	—	—
13	London	1889	March	about 24	8	0	—	Fish	—
14	London	1889	May	about 11	4	1	Pork	Pig	—
15	London	1889	August	about 5	5	0	Beef	Ox	—
16	Manchester	1894	November	—	160	3	Milk	Cow	Gaertner.
17	London	1895	June	about 12	3	0	Meat pies	Ox	—
18	Mansfield	1896	February	12–24 for most	265	0	Potted meat	Ox and Pig	(Inconclusive.)
19	Atherton	1898	—	1–2	—	—	Pickled tongues	Ox	—
20	Hatton	1898	—	—	185	1	Veal pies	Calf	B. suipestifer.
21	Salford	1898	June	about 6–12	5	1	Cold hashed beef	Ox	B. suipestifer (from serum reactions).

No.	Place	Year	Month	Incubation	Cases	Deaths	Food	Animal	Organism
22	Chadderton (and Oldham)	1898	July	Most 6–7; 3–29 as extremes	47	4	Veal pies	Calf	B. suipestifer.
23	Surbiton	1898	August	8–44	10	2	Fresh ox tongue (also ribs of lamb)	Ox	B. suipestifer.
24	Nuneaton	1899	April	5½–48½	42	0	Chitterlings	Pig	—
25	Greenwich (London)	1899	July	—	about 100	0	Milk	Cow	—
26	Sheffield	1899	November	1–3½	24	1	Corned beef	Ox	B. enteritidis.
27	Rochdale	1900	August	—	141	0	Ice-cream	—	—
28	Cressage (Salop)	1900	September	3–5	7	2	Goose gravy and giblets	Goose	—
29	London (Islington)	1901	July	—	4	1	Cream (in jar)	—	—
30	London (City)	1902	July	Within a few hours	17	0	Ice-cream	—	—
31	London (Fulham)	1902	September	—	4	1	Stewed rabbit, warmed up	Rabbit	B. suipestifer.
32	Derby	1902	September	4–24	221 +	1	Pork pies	Pig	Gaertner*.
33	Battersea	1904	July	8–14	64 +	0	Ice-cream	—	(Inconclusive.)
34	Birmingham	1905	July	½–8½	52	0	Ice-cream	—	(Inconclusive.)
35	Eastbourne	1905	October	—	about 60	0	Brawn	Pig	—
36	Accrington	1906	Jan.–Feb.	12–36	50	0	Brawn	Pig	Gaertner.
37	Partick	1906	May	1–4	12	0	Tinned beef	Ox	Gaertner (from serum reaction).
38	Sculcoates Workhouse	1906	June	—	35	6	Frozen meat	—	—
39	Bedford	1906	June	8–16	29	0	Pork pie	Pig	Gaertner.
40	Wigan	1907	January	—	168 +	0	Potted tongues	Ox and pig	Gaertner.
41	Tunstall	1907	April	10–14	3	1	Tinned salmon	Salmon	—
42	Partick	1907	June	about 24	3	0	"Hough and potted chicken"	—	B. enteritidis.
43	Ashton-under-Lyne	1907	August	4–17	44 +	0	Udder	Cow	—

* Available information insufficient to state the precise Gaertner sub-group. This applies to each instance when "Gaertner" is used in the Tables.

TABLE I.—BRITISH OUTBREAKS—*continued.*

Number	Place	Year	Month	Incubation period (in hours)	Number of Cases	Deaths	Kind of food eaten	Animal from which derived	Bacteria isolated
44	Longton	1907	August	12–24	4	1	Tinned salmon	Salmon	B. enteritidis.
45	Tollesbury	1907	September	1½–4	80	0	Brawn	Pig	B. enteritidis.
46	Murrow	1908	May	12–48	18	3	Brawn	Pig	B. suipestifer.
47	St Annes-on-the-Sea	1908	July	2–12	76	3	Potted beef (34 cases) / Pork pies (42 cases)	Ox / Pig	} Gaertner.
48	Whitefield	1908	July	—	11	0	Pork pies	Pig	—
49	Newcastle-under-Lyme	1908	July	6–12	31	0	Milk	Cow	B. coli.
50	Hornsey	1908	July	—	6	1	—	Shrimps	Gaertner.
51	Bakewell	1908	August	1–16	30 +	2	Milk	Cow	—
52	Mossley	1908	August	—	7	0	Beef pies	Ox	Gaertner.
53	Blackpool	1908	September	—	29	1	Pork pies	Pig	—
54	Wirksworth	1908	September	—	—	1	Beef brawn	Ox	Gaertner.
55	Disley and Marple	1908	October	—	about 50	1	Brawn	Cow	—
56	Aberdeen	1908	November	—	—	0	Milk	Cow	—
57	Limerick	1909	May	3–9	73	9	Beef	Ox	B. enteritidis.
58	Nuneaton	1909	June	2–6	67	9	Ice-cream	—	Gaertner.
59	Banff	1909	June	8–13	16	0	Tinned corned beef	Ox	—
60	London	1909	July		7	0	Steak and kidney pie	Ox	B. coli, etc. (no Gaertner).
61	Bristol	1909	August	Within 12 hrs.	54 +	0	Corned beef	Ox	(Inconclusive.)
62	Kensington	1910	April	—	8	0	Sausages (from the sausage casings)	—	—
63	Downham	1910	May	1–5	18 +	0	Brawn	Pig	Gaertner.
64	Warwick	1910	June	20 or more for most	20 +	1	Boiled (fresh) beef	Ox	—
65	St Helens	1910	August	2–10 (3–6 hrs. for most)	32	0	Tinned corned beef	Ox	(Inconclusive.)
66	Astley	1910	August	Within 1 hour	7	0	Tinned tongue	?	—
67	Burslem	1910	August	7–8	4	1	Tinned salmon	Salmon	—
68	Castle Bromwich	1910	August	--	12	1	Ice-cream	—	—

No.	Place	Year	Month	Interval between meal and illness (hrs.)	No. affected	Deaths	Food	Animal	Organism
69	Wrexham	1910	August	5–45 (12 hrs. for most)	107	5	Pork pies	Pig	B. paratyphosus B (B. suipestifer). (Inconclusive.)
70	Norbiton	1910	August	All within ½ hour	80–100	o	Fish, potatoes, oil	—	—
71	Stretford	1910	September	—	20	o	Braised beef	Ox	} (Inconclusive.)
72	Rowley Regis	1910	October	—	20–30	o	{ Cold boiled beef, Cold boiled ham	Ox, Pig	}
73	Ramsgate	1910	October	1–3	30 +	o	Sausage rolls	—	—
74	Saltley (Birmingham)	1910	December	—	4	1	Kippers	Herring	—
75	Bingham	1910	March	½–6	—	o	Brawn	Pig	B. enteritidis (from serum reactions).
76	Chester	1911		—	10	o	Corned beef	Ox	(Inconclusive.) No Gaertner.
77	Warrington	1911	April	9–16	23	o	Brawn	Pig	Gaertner.
78	Edinburgh	1911	June	—	About 100	—	Milk	Cow	B. suipestifer.
79	Chesterfield	1911	June	—	168	1	Pork pies	Pig	Gaertner.
80	Bacup	1911	June	4–20	213 +	4	Brawn, roast pork (from same pigs)	Pig	—
81	Clapham	1911	July	6–9	8	1	Pineapple jelly	—	—
82	Walthamstow	1911	September	—	7 +	1	Tinned tongue	—	(Inconclusive).
83	Wigan	1911	September	2	11	o	Corned beef	Ox	B. enteritidis.
84	Bacup	1912	October	9–24 (average 14)	38	o	Roast leg of pork	Pig	Gaertner.
85	Eccles	1912	May	—	19	o	Pressed veal	Calf	—
86	Chorley	1912	May	8–14	241	o	Pork pies	Pig	Gaertner.
87	Treviscoe (Cornwall)	1912	July	—	57	o	Meat (ham, fowl, beef?)	?	—
88	Manchester	1912	October	5–55 (10–40 for most)	163	3	Chitterlings	Pig	Gaertner.
89	Northwich	1913	May	3–4	14	o	Home pressed beef	Ox	—
90	Newcastle-upon-Tyne	1913	October, November	—	523	o	Milk	Cow	B. enteritidis.
91	Skelmanthorpe	1914	February	—	5	1	Tinned corned beef	Ox	Gaertner.

TABLE I.—British Outbreaks—*continued.*

Number	Place	Year	Month	Incubation period (in hours)	Number of Cases	Deaths	Kind of food eaten	Animal from which derived	Bacteria isolated
92	Colne	1914	May	—	3	3	Possibly mutton	? sheep	—
93	Cambridge	1914	May	4–72	95	0	Fresh salmon	Salmon	—
94	Todmorden	1914	July	—	3	2	Fresh potted meat	?	—
95	Withnell and Chorley	1914	July	—	317	2	Milk	Cow	B. enteritidis.
96	Oswestry	1914	July	15–36	86	0	Boiled pork pressed†	Pig	Gaertner.
97	Tamworth	1914	July	—	27	0	Pork	Pig	B. enteritidis.
98	Newcastle-under-Lyme	1914	October	Most less than 12 hours	468	2	Milk	Cow	B. enteritidis.
99	Westminster (London)	1914	August	—	10	1	Rice cooked in fat	—	Indefinite.
100	Liverpool	1915	January	—	18	0	Canned peaches	Salmon	—
101	Bradford	1915	April	—	3	1	Tinned salmon	Salmon	—
102	Newport (Mon.)	1915	May	12–24 for most	75	2	Brawn	Pig	B. aertrycke.
103	Leeds	1915	May	2–39 (5–12 for most)	154	1	Pork pies	Pig	Gaertner.
104	Bacup	1915	June	6–24	66	0	Stuffed roast pork	Pig	B. enteritidis.
105	Frome	1916	July	3–16	6	1	Beefsteak pudding	Ox	B. enteritidis (toxins).
106	Cambridge	1917	July	4–15	61	—	Chicken and sauce	Fowl	B. enteritidis.
107	Glasgow	1917	November	—		1	Potatoes	—	—
108	Brighton	1917	November	—	28	2	Fried fish	Ling and cod	B. enteritidis.
109	Trowbridge	1918	January	9–30	47	2	Chitterlings	Pig	B. suipestifer.
110	Tamworth	1918	February	$\frac{1}{2}$–5	10	0	Tinned pressed beef	Ox	—
111	Bordon	1918	February	5–48	102	0	Tinned salmon	Salmon	—
112	Bradford	1918	April	—	1	0	Tinned herrings	Herring	Gaertner.

† Really a brawn, only with large pieces of meat, and included as such in the summary.

ADDENDUM II.

ANIMAL DISEASES CAUSED BY INFECTION WITH MEMBERS
OF THE GAERTNER GROUP OF BACILLI.

1. *Swine fever.* This disease is now generally accepted as due to a
filterable virus, but in a considerable proportion of cases *B. suipestifer*, a
member of the Gaertner group, is also found to be present, not as a mere
passive concomitant but apparently with a distinct, although subsidiary,
disease-producing rôle. The proportion of cases of swine fever in which
this bacillus is found seems to vary from 0 to 45 per cent. or over (Uhlenhuth, Hübener, Xylander and Bohtz (1908), Uhlenhuth and Haendel
(1913), Grabert (1907)).

While recorded investigations give the occurrence of this bacillus as
prevalent to the considerable extent indicated, it is of importance to note
that in many of the records the term *B. suipestifer* is used in a wide sense
and includes many organisms which with any strict definition of the Gaertner
group, such as should be employed, must be excluded as not members of
it. Uhlenhuth and Haendel (1913) discuss at some length the varieties of
B. suipestifer and while they point out that many of these are culturally
identical and differ chiefly as regards virulence, motility and other variable
characters, yet they include under this term, as varieties, organisms described by Dorset and also by Joest and Grabert which do not ferment
glucose, and the bacillus described by Rietsch and Jobert from swine fever
pigs at Marseilles which produced acid and clot in milk. Also the eight
bacterial strains described by Uhlenhuth, Hübener, Xylander and Bohtz
(1908) which failed to be agglutinated must be regarded as suspicious,
although they report them as culturally in agreement with *B. suipestifer*,
since they do not appear to have recognized the existence of para-Gaertner
organisms. (The dulcite and salicin tests for example were not employed.)

Dammann and Stedefeder (1910) in an outbreak at Voldagsen isolated a
bacillus (*B. voldagsen*) which caused an infectious disease in pigs, and Glässer
isolated an identical or almost identical organism (*B. glässer*) from another
outbreak. These authors considered them to be true causal organisms
of a variety of swine fever (Ferkel typhus), but the current German view
appears to be that they are variants of *B. suipestifer* occurring in cases of
hog-cholera (Schweinepest). Culturally they differ from *B. suipestifer* in
several important points, particularly in producing permanent acidity in
milk, and in not fermenting glucose to the extent of gas production.
Culturally they stand between *B. typhosus* and *B. suipestifer*. They are
only slightly pathogenic and are only influenced in trifling degree by
B suipestifer immune serum.

It should be stated that considerable differences of opinion still exist
amongst authorities as to what exactly constitutes swine fever. Schern
and Stange (1914), for example, classify into three groups:

(*a*) Schweinepest caused by *B. suipestifer*—classical swine fever.

(*b*) Schweinepest caused by *B. suipestifer* and a filterable virus. Mixed
infection.

(*c*) A disease of hogs characterised by a haemorrhagic septicaemia;

caused by the filterable virus and not identical with the classical Schweine-pest.

In one of the most recent investigations, that of Gildemeister and Baerthlein (1915), ten *B. suipestifer* strains obtained from diseased swine inoculated in Germany with an American swine fever virus were culturally all alike and agreed with the true Gaertner type but the differentiating tests were insufficient as they did not employ salicin, raffinose, saccharose or dulcite. Their agglutination results, however, suggest that these strains were closely allied to *B. voldagsen* and *B. glässer*. The importance of these variants in human pathology is unknown, but outbreaks have been described by Bernhardt and by Neukirch.

Bernhardt (1913) describes a small outbreak of food poisoning, with one death, after eating the meat of a necessity slaughtered cow. From the organs of the fatal case he isolated a bacillus of the Gaertner type which only differed culturally in that it failed to ferment glucose in twenty-four hours, and only produced a little gas after forty-eight hours. It, however, produced alkali in milk like the ordinary type and unlike the Glässer-Voldagsen strains. This bacillus was not agglutinated by *B. enteritidis* or *B. paratyphoid B* sera, but was agglutinated to the titre limit by a *B. voldagsen* serum. The sera of the patients agglutinated this strain but not *B. enteritidis* and only two showed a positive reaction with *B. paratyphosus B*, and this in very low dilution (1 in 20). Bernhardt isolated the Voldagsen-Glässer bacillus from three other outbreaks in each instance from a fatal case, and some of these strains failed to ferment glucose at all. The sugar-alcohol tests used were not extensive and it is not clear that at least some of the strains were not the ordinary type of *B. suipestifer*.

Neukirch (1918) has described an extensive outbreak in Anatolia and Constantinople in 1915 amongst men in which the cases were of a typhoid-septic or dysenteric type with a mortality of about 50 per cent. From a large proportion of the cases he isolated bacilli of the Gaertner group type, and which from his serological tests he considered to be closely related to the Glässer-Voldagsen type. An examination of his cultural reactions, however, throws considerable doubt upon this relationship since the strains fermented glucose with gas formation (but slower than *B. paratyphosus B*) while they gave the typical acid followed by rapid alkali production in litmus milk characteristic of the true Gaertner strains. It is more probable that the outbreak was a very severe one of *B. paratyphosus B* infection.

In Scotland McGowan (1915) carried out some very thorough post-mortem investigations on cases of swine fever. Cultures were made from the various organs and lesions of eleven cases of this disease in the neigh-bourhood of Edinburgh and twenty-seven organisms were isolated. None of them however belong to the true Gaertner group as shown by their action upon glucose, dulcite, and litmus milk, while all (with one possible exception) were non-motile. In two other isolated cases true *B. suipestifer* was not found.

McGowan (1917) in a subsequent report records the bacteriological findings in four further outbreaks in three separate piggeries. Although the bacteriological examinations were very thorough and included the examination of many different organs from eighty-five pigs, organisms resembling *B. suipestifer* were found in two cases only, i.e. from the duo-denum of one pig (pig 1) and from the heart blood, duodenum and intestine of another animal (pig 4). These strains were culturally fully identical with *B. suipestifer* including the fermentation of dulcite and sorbite (both gas and acid), and alkali production in litmus milk. None of the other organisms could be classed as Gaertner group organisms. *B. suisepticus*, on the other hand, was found in a large proportion of the pigs.

Eberson (1915) studied the chief groups of organisms found in a number of hogs artificially infected with the hog-cholera virus, fifty-five animals being examined: 106 so-called paratyphoid strains were isolated. The cultural character of these organisms are not given in detail, but for some the few cultural tests employed show clearly that they are not true Gaertner strains while for the rest the tests employed are totally inadequate to say if they are Gaertner organisms or not. Yet in this paper it is set out that "classification of the organisms shows that the greatest number belonged to the paratyphosus B group."

It is, in the writer's opinion, a fair and justifiable criticism to make that if more exact and extended cultural investigations were made of the organisms present in pigs suffering from swine fever a considerably smaller percentage would be recorded as true *B. suipestifer* strains. Apart, however, from such necessary corrections it would still appear to be true that genuine Gaertner organisms are frequently met with in cases of swine fever, that is organisms which with the most refined bacteriological tests are indistinguishable from the strains isolated from human victims of food poisoning.

2. *Septicaemia and other diseases of calves.* It would appear that while calf septicaemia, dysentery and pneumonia are caused by a number of different bacteria, in a certain proportion of cases Gaertner group bacilli are either the cause or are found to be present.

Thomassen (1897) described a fatal septicaemia in calves in the neighbourhood of Utrecht and isolated a bacillus, now identified with *B. enteritidis* from the spleens, kidneys and other organs of the affected animals. Since that date Gaertner group bacilli have been reported by several continental observers in cases of septicaemia, white scour, etc. Such reports have been published by Zeller (1909), Titze and Weichel (1909), Schmidt (1907), Riemer (1908) and Winzer (1911).

Several continental investigators have reported the occurrence of necrotic areas in the spleen, liver and other organs of calves in slaughter-houses. These were first investigated by Langer (1904), who isolated from them a bacillus which he called *B. nodulifaciens bovis*, but which was shown by Pitt (1909) and later observers to be a true Gaertner group organism. Pitt found that the calves frequently came from the same place and the same stalls and probably therefore represent the results of endemic infection. Ledschbor (1909) and also Joest (1914) and others have found similar bacilli.

Uhlenhuth and Hübener have shown that Jensen's paracolon bacillus, described by him as the cause of calf dysentery, is in at least many cases a true Gaertner group bacillus. Jensen's (1913) own figures however show that Gaertner group infections are only responsible for a small proportion of the cases which he groups under the term "Kalbërruhr." Of 251 cases he only found these bacilli in sixteen or 6·4 per cent. Apparently they were all in new born calves and no doubt were all infected at parturition. It is possible that a few may be of human origin but this is a most unlikely source of infection, and the most probable origin is either an infected cow or infected litter, etc.

On the other hand, Meyer, Traum and Roadhouse (1916) describe *B. enteritidis* as the cause of a severe outbreak of infectious diarrhoea or scour occurring amongst calves at the Agricultural Experiment Station, California.

Zschiesche (1918) has recently called attention to the heavy mortality from calves in East Prussia from diarrhoea conditions similar to those described by Jensen. He ascribes many of these cases to bacilli of the Gaertner group, but his results are very incompletely recorded so that it is not possible to say to what extent the bacilli isolated from the 176 calves examined are genuine Gaertner group organisms. The fact that these Gaertner group bacilli isolated from calves can set up human disease is illustrated by the case recorded by Meyer (see p. 73).

3. *Pyaemic and septicaemic conditions in the domestic animals generally.* Bollinger in 1876 first drew attention to the frequency of the association of food poisoning outbreaks in man with the consumption of the meat of animals suffering from such diseases. In a certain number of cases Gaertner group bacilli have been isolated from such conditions and apart from food poisoning outbreaks. For example the *B. morbificans bovis* of Basenau is a Gaertner organism and was isolated by him from a cow emergency slaughtered on account of puerperal metritis, while Fisher in 1896 isolated *B. enteritidis* from the spleen of a cow with udder inflammation. Also of particular interest is the outbreak of acute mastitis in cows recorded by Zwick (1909) and Zwick and Weichel (1910) in which Gaertner group bacilli were isolated from two out of twenty-one cases.

Against these recorded cases we have the fact that a long series of bacteriological examinations of animals suffering from septicaemic diseases —made on the continent—have failed to show Gaertner group bacilli, except in rare instances.

We must therefore conclude that while conditions of this sort may be caused by Gaertner group bacilli it is a rare and exceptional occurrence and the vast proportion of cases are due to the ordinary pathogenic pyogenic bacteria.

4. *Enteritis in cows.* Such cases are of exceptional interest in view of the fact that in a number of meat poisoning outbreaks the meat has been derived from a cow suffering from enteritis. Instances of enteritis in cows, unassociated with food poisoning outbreaks, in which Gaertner group bacilli have been isolated are rare and the writer has only been able to find the following.

Mohler and Buckley (1902) record an outbreak in which seven out of twenty-one cows in a cowshed suffered from enteritis and died, while three others exhibited early symptoms but recovered. A Gaertner group bacillus was isolated from all the fatal cases. One cow apparently recovered from the acute attack, but ultimately died twenty-six days after the onset.

Meissner, Berge and Kohlstock (1912) describe an interesting outbreak. Dysentery was prevalent amongst some calves, causing the death of some although the majority recovered. One of these animals which had apparently recovered was transferred to pasture land shared by a number of cows. A number of these then suffered from diarrhoea and enteritis and died. The only one investigated showed *B. enteritidis* in pure culture. The affected cows were then moved to cow stalls. These contained two lame cows and a 1½ year old bull, none of which had been out in the pasture field. One of these two cows fell ill after the addition of the affected cows and from it *B. enteritidis* was isolated. The calf, which had apparently recovered and which was transferred to the field, was then examined bacteriologically and *B. enteritidis* isolated (the report does not say from which organs). A further calf which had died of enteritis was also subsequently examined and *B. enteritidis* isolated. In this outbreak we have an illustration of a calf suffering from a Gaertner group infection recovering and acting as a carrier of infection.

5. *Abortion in mares.* While it is evident in the great majority of cases that this condition, at least in this country, is due to bacteria other than food poisoning bacilli (see *Annual Report* (1914) of Chief Veterinary Officer of the Board of Agriculture) there is evidence that in certain outbreaks bacilli of the Gaertner group are present in the lesions and in a number of cases have been reported as the cause of the condition. In 1893 Kilborne and Smith studied an abortion outbreak occurring amongst the mares of a large stud in Pennsylvania and isolated a bacillus which they grouped as a hog-cholera bacillus. The characters described are insufficient to group it as undeniably a true Gaertner group organism, but it fermented glucose but not lactose and saccharose, and the other characteristics given are those of Gaertner organisms.

Similar bacilli have been isolated from American outbreaks by Good and Corbett, and by Meyer and Boerner (1913). The latter observers from an outbreak in 1913 in Pennsylvania isolated a bacillus which they called *B. abortus equi*. The serum of the aborting animals gave positive agglutination results as high as 1 : 2500 with this bacillus, but a complete complement fixation with comparatively high titres was only noted in four animals. This bacillus exhibited the cultural characters of the Gaertner strains except that the growth on agar slope was membranous, dry and brittle, and the gas produced in dulcite media was large in amount. One of the two strains isolated by Good also exhibited similar characteristics on agar. Their agglutination results suggest that their *B. abortus equi* is neither *B. enteritidis* nor *B. paratyphosus B*, while it was only partially in agreement with the only strain of *B. suipestifer* tested. The authors put it in a separate sub-group.

Meissner and Berge (1917) isolated what they call *B. paratyphosus B* forty-five times from the organs of fifty-seven foetuses (four to eight months old). The sera of the mares agglutinated the bacteria isolated in dilutions of 1 : 1000 to 1 : 2000 and in some cases in higher dilution, while normal serum was only agglutinated 1 to 300. These bacteria were also agglutinated by *B. paratyphosus B* serum.

In 1897 Lignières and in 1905 Lignières and Zabala isolated a Gaertner group bacillus from a series of cases of epizootic abortion in mares, sheep and cows in France and Argentina. In Holland outbreaks ascribed to members of this group have been described by de Jong, and by Van Heelsbergen (1914). The bacillus isolated by Van Heelsbergen was pathogenic to the smaller laboratory animals and, as far as its cultural characters were tested, agreed with the Gaertner group. The agglutination reactions seem to show that it is not identical with either *B. enteritidis*, *B. suipestifer*, or *B. paratyphosus B*.

Good and Corbett (1913) isolated a very similar bacillus from the placenta, foetuses and uterine exudates in six different studs. Their bacillus agglutinated the sera of infected animals in dilutions of from 1 : 500 to 1 : 5000 but was affected by normal horse sera only in low dilutions. The serum of an animal immunized against this bacillus failed to agglutinate either *B. enteritidis* or *B. cholera suis*.

With their bacillus they succeeded in causing abortion in a ewe and a sow by intravenous and in guinea-pigs by subcutaneous injections, the organism being recovered from the uterine exudates. An injection of 2 c.c. of an agar emulsion into a pregnant mare caused abortion with the typical symptoms of the natural infection, while the organism was found in abundance in the internal organs of the foetus, as well as from the foetal membranes and uterus of the mare.

The writer is not concerned with the question as to how far these bacilli were the true cause of the abortion and other symptoms or whether they played a rôle analogous to that of *B. suipestifer* in swine fever, but their presence in this condition in horses is certainly of considerable interest.

6. *Certain diseases of birds.* Epidemics, usually marked by a high fatality rate, have been recorded as affecting a number of different species of birds and from which Gaertner group bacilli have been isolated. The best known are the outbreaks in parrots, the so-called Psittacosis disease (see *Baumgarten's Jahresbericht*, 1896, for an account of several outbreaks). Nocard in 1893 isolated a bacillus, which he called *B. psittacosis*, from the bone marrow of birds which had died on the journey from Buenos Ayres. In subsequent epidemics this bacillus has been isolated both from the diseased parrots and from the blood of the human cases. From the parrots the disease has spread to man, and in April, 1892, an extensive outbreak occurred in Paris, with forty-two known cases and fourteen deaths.

B. psittacosis is undoubtedly a Gaertner group organism probably identical with *B. suipestifer* (Böhme, 1906, Selter, 1916). Tartakowsky has described an infectious enteritis in sparrows due to a Gaertner bacillus.

Joest (1907) isolated a bacillus, apparently a Gaertner group organism, from a canary suffering, with others, from an epidemic disease associated with catarrhal enteritis and splenic tumour. Zingle (1914) in 1913 isolated in pure culture a Gaertner group organism from pigeons in an outbreak affecting fourteen birds in the military pigeon station at Strassburg. This strain was agglutinated nearly to the titre limit by a *B. paratyphosus* B serum but was only partially agglutinated by a *B. enteritidis* serum, so apparently it is the former organism, according to German nomenclature. Manninger (1913) investigated three birds of the finch family sent to him from the Buda-Pest Zoological Gardens and isolated from them a Gaertner group bacillus. The birds suffered from an acute intestinal catarrh. Like the bacillus from the last outbreak this organism was only agglutinated in moderate degree by a *B. enteritidis* serum but to the titre limit by a *B. paratyphosus* B serum.

The outbreak of acute infectious disease in young pheasants recorded by Klein (1893) in which over 700 out of 1800 died may have been due to a Gaertner strain, but the characters of the bacillus isolated from the heart blood are insufficient to settle this point and the fact that indol is said to have been produced is against this assumption.

7. *Canine distemper.* The writer has only come across one report dealing with the presence of Gaertner bacilli in dogs. Torrey and Rahl (1912), in a series of sixty-three consecutive cases of natural and experimental distemper, isolated *B. enteritidis* in one or more of the internal organs in twelve cases (19 per cent.). They suggest the bacilli invaded the organs in the final stages since 75 per cent. of the findings were in animals

severely attacked. The bacilli were non-toxic to dogs. Their characters are not given in detail but were said to be identical in cultural and agglutination characters with *B. enteritidis* (Gaertner).

8. *Diseases amongst rodents*. *B. typhi murium* (a Gaertner group organism) was isolated by Löffler as the cause of an epidemic in mice and has been isolated subsequently from other mice epidemics. It has been used as living poison to set up an epizootic among mice and so cause their extermination. In the same way a number of Gaertner group bacilli have been used to set up infective disease in rats. Of these Danysz's bacillus is the best known.

Spontaneous outbreaks of infectious disease amongst rats and mice and due to Gaertner group strains are not uncommon. Three such have occurred at widely different periods amongst the writer's laboratory mice. Extensive outbreaks amongst laboratory guinea-pigs due to these bacilli are not at all uncommon (O'Brien and others).

A number of similar outbreaks in rats or mice have been recorded on the continent, while Pappenheimer and Wedel (1914) have described an epidemic in America due to a strain which agreed in every respect with the Liverpool rat virus.

Davies, Heaven and Walker Hall (1917) have described a very extensive rat epizootic on board a ship from Buenos Ayres due to *B. suipestifer* or a very closely allied variety.

Outbreaks of disease in other animals may possibly have been due to Gaertner group bacilli, but the bacilli have not been sufficiently worked out. Mori (1905), for example, describes a bacillus isolated from a cat, which, with several others, had died from an epizootic in Siena. The characters given are insufficient to indicate whether it was a Gaertner organism or not. In several food poisoning outbreaks due to Gaertner group bacilli cats eating the incriminated food have been affected and made seriously ill.

9. In connection with the problem of the extent to which Gaertner group bacilli are responsible for disease in domestic animals some results obtained by the writer (Savage, 1918 a) are of interest. The sera of a number of domestic animals passed as healthy were examined and, in a considerable proportion of them, specific agglutinins were present against one or other member of the Gaertner group. The following summary gives the results of 133 examinations. In this table a positive reaction with a dilution of 1 : 20 only is classed as negative; a "slight" reaction is a positive reaction with a dilution of 1 : 50 with any one of the three organisms (*B. enteritidis*, *B. suipestifer*, *B. paratyphosus B*), while a "marked" reaction comprises a positive reaction with any one of these three organisms in a dilution of 1 : 100 or above.

Animal	Number examined	Percentages		
		No reaction	Slight reaction	Marked reaction
Calf	14	100	—	—
Cow and Ox	26	11	35	54
Sheep	18	78	11	11
Pig	36	39	19	42
Horse	39	41	33	26

These agglutinins were absent in all the calves, were mostly absent from sheep, but were fairly well developed in 40 to 50 per cent. of the pigs,

cows and oxen examined. They were also present in a considerable proportion of the horses tested. The failure to demonstrate these agglutinins
in the calf and their definite development in many of the cows and oxen
sera suggest that they are not present in the new born animal but develop
later in life. The available data is insufficient to enable a definite opinion
to be given as to whether these positive reactions with Gaertner strains
are to be ascribed to an old infection with these bacilli, but they suggest
this possibility.

ADDENDUM III.

DISTRIBUTION OF GAERTNER GROUP BACILLI IN NATURE APART FROM PATHOLOGICAL CONDITIONS.

The distribution of these bacilli in nature is of such great significance in
connection with the problems of food poisoning, and many of the results
have been so conflicting, that it is necessary to give in some detail particulars
of the investigations carried out in this connection. The data is conveniently grouped as follows: in the human intestine, in the animal intestine, in foodstuffs, particularly prepared meats.

A. In the human intestine.

B. paratyphosus B is found in the intestine in cases of paratyphoid fever
and in persons who have comparatively recently had an attack of paratyphoid fever and are acting as acute or chronic carriers.

Apart from these cases all the English investigators have failed to find
that *B. paratyphosus B* or other true Gaertner group organisms are natural
inhabitants of the healthy human intestine.

In 1907–9 the writer (Savage, 1907, 1908 *a*) examined very carefully
and by methods of proved utility fifty-three specimens of human excreta
from healthy persons or from persons suffering from disease, a few being
cases of paratyphoid fever. Apart from finding *B. paratyphosus B* in actual
cases of that disease only one organism of the true Gaertner group was
isolated; this was a *B. enteritidis*.

Morgan (1906) examined about 300 cases of summer diarrhoea and only
found two true Gaertner organisms, both *B. suipestifer*.

Williams, Murray and Rundle (1910) examined the stools of 100 normal
children and failed to find any true Gaertner group organisms.

Bainbridge and O'Brien (1911) examined the faeces and urine of numerous
typhoid convalescents and failed to isolate any true Gaertner group bacilli.

Lewis (1911) examined 214 specimens of faeces from 146 normal children
and seventy specimens of faeces from sixty-one cases of diarrhoea in
infants. Only *one* strain identical with true Gaertner group bacilli was
isolated. It was pathogenic but the precise sub-group was not determined.

The German results are conflicting. Conradi, Prigge and Sachsmüke
(1909) and others recorded *B. paratyphosus B* as present in the excreta of
a considerable proportion of typhoid convalescents and healthy persons,
while Seiffert (1909), Sobernheim (1910), Aumann, Tiberti (1911) and others
do not confirm these observations.

Aumann's (1911) figures include 799 specimens of human excreta, urine, blood or vomit examined in the Municipal Hamburg Hygienic Institute, 1905–1910. Of these 498 were excreta specimens and 6 per cent. (thirty-one specimens) showed true Gaertner group bacilli, thirteen being paratyphoid bacilli and eighteen *B. enteritidis*. In all but one the presence of these bacilli was closely associated with epidemics or cases of disease. In the 301 other specimens three paratyphoid *B* bacilli were isolated, in each instance from a case of paratyphoid fever.

B. In the animal intestine.

a. Animals used for food. In view of the fact that faecal contamination of food during and sometimes after preparation is common, it becomes of cardinal importance to ascertain to what extent bacilli of the Gaertner group occur in the intestines of healthy animals. The domestic animals used for food are naturally the most important in this connection.

The results obtained may be divided into three distinct phases. We have first the earlier German reports which supported the conception that these bacilli were natural intestinal inhabitants, then independently of these but in part carried out concurrently the investigations in this country which quite failed to support this contention, and lastly a series of recent investigations in Germany and elsewhere which support the English results.

Uhlenhuth, Hübener, Xylander and Bohtz (1908) investigated bacteriologically the intestinal contents of 600 pigs from the Central Berlin slaughterhouse. Although they only examined one loopful of the intestinal contents, they isolated *B. suipestifer* from 8·4 per cent. (fifty-one cases) of the animals.

In confirmation of these results Seiffert (1909) found the bacilli twice in sixty pigs, Ecker in four out of ten pigs and Grabert in seven out of twenty-three pigs.

The cultural tests which these investigators employed, and which were accepted by them as sufficient, are not adequate to distinguish the bacilli from the para-Gaertner bacilli which not infrequently are present in the healthy animal gut. These investigators for example did not test the fermentation properties of their organisms upon dulcite, salicin or saccharose.

Some virulence tests—subcutaneous inoculation of mice—were performed and the mice succumbed. The strains were agglutinated by hog-cholera sera but the exact dilutions employed are not given.

In healthy calves and sheep Uhlenhuth, Hübener and Andreijew found organisms in small numbers which were possibly paratyphoid bacilli. Andreijew (1910) is also frequently credited with finding true Gaertner bacilli in sheep intestines, but what he did find was bacilli "which in their cultural and biological characters could be, with more or less probability, added to the hog-cholera group of bacilli." Para-Gaertner bacilli are not uncommon in sheep.

On the other hand, there are a number of negative German findings. For example, Titze and Weichel (1909) examined the excreta of forty-four cattle, sixty calves, fifteen sheep, three goats, sixteen dogs, twenty-four rabbits, fifty guinea-pigs, thirteen fowls, fourteen pigeons, six geese and fourteen sparrows with quite negative results except that in the excreta of one horse they found a paratyphoid bacillus.

Ecker also examined the intestinal contents of twelve horses, sixteen cattle, eight sheep, one goat and five rats, and only in the case of one horse did he find a true Gaertner group bacillus.

Horn and Huber (1912) examined the intestinal content of 100 healthy animals without finding any true Gaertner group bacilli although they found some allied forms.

Aumann examined the excreta of 200 recently slaughtered animals, consisting of 101 pigs, forty-eight cattle, forty-one sheep and ten calves, and failed to find true Gaertner group bacilli in any of them.

Only a few English investigations appear to have been carried out, but their results are entirely opposed to the view that these organisms are natural intestinal inhabitants.

Morgan (1905) examined the faeces and intestinal contents of a number of animals and isolated twenty-one cultures of bacilli of the Gaertner type. They were, however, not isolated by direct cultivation from the intestinal contents but only from animals inoculated with the material under examination, a method which is now admitted to be unreliable for this purpose.

In 1906–1908 the writer examined with great care (for example over 700 plates were inoculated) the intestinal contents of twenty-six animals and five specimens of animal excreta, the animals selected being seven pigs, six bullocks or cows, five calves, four sheep, eight horses and one mouse. No true Gaertner group organisms could be found, although a considerable number of para-Gaertner bacilli were isolated which culturally resembled true Gaertner bacilli extremely closely.

These results have been confirmed by Bainbridge (1911) who examined the intestinal contents of fifty pigs without finding any true Gaertner group bacilli.

In a later examination the writer (Savage, 1918) examined some of the internal organs of thirty-six healthy pigs and ten calves without finding any true Gaertner group organisms.

As mentioned above quite recent continental and American investigations substantiate the views of the author as shown by the following reports.

Fischer (1915) examined eighty-five old calves, ten young calves and ten adult oxen without finding any Gaertner bacilli.

Christiansen (1917) examined thirty-four calves without finding any true bacilli of this group. One closely allied bacillus (a para-Gaertner strain) was isolated and this author remarks that he frequently found this organism in older calves. It was non-pathogenic.

Trawinski (1917) examined the intestinal contents of 500 healthy pigs and from them isolated twenty-six strains which he included in the Gaertner group. The pigs came from a district where there had been no epidemics and were kept under observation for eight to ten days in the slaughterhouse. Further cultural investigation of these strains divided them into three groups. The eight members of one group although they fermented dulcite failed to ferment sorbite and produced indol. Another group of sixteen strains also produced indol and failed to ferment either sorbite or dulcite. Only the two strains in the remaining group were culturally identical with the recognized pathogenic members of the group. His agglutination and absorption tests confirm the cultural reactions except that the eight organisms of the first group serologically showed a relationship to B. aertrycke and to B. suipestifer. While therefore without the application of certain essential cultural tests 5 per cent. of Gaertner group organisms were obtained, this was reduced to 0·4 per cent. when more detailed cultural examinations were employed.

Russ and Trawinski (1918) examined 1000 strains from horse manure and while seventy-seven (7·7 per cent.) were of the Gaertner group type closer study showed that only two strains were culturally quite identical with the true Gaertner organisms, while a further five strains only differed in that they failed to ferment rhamnose. Salicin was not employed, while none of the organisms were agglutinated by *B. enteritidis* or *B. paratyphosus B* serum.

Jordan (1918 *a*), in America, examined the intestinal contents of 291 normal swine, investigating in all 1419 strains. No organism was isolated which had the recognized characters of true Gaertner group bacilli, while this was confirmed by their failure to show any agglutination affinities with these organisms.

Summing up the matter it seems a reliable deduction that the Gaertner group of organisms are not natural inhabitants of the intestine or other organs of domestic animals and the earlier German work is unreliable and is probably to be explained by failure to use a sufficient series of differentiating tests, para-Gaertner organisms (which are not uncommon) being confused with the true strains.

β. *Rats and mice.* Apart from animals used for animal food, evidence has been adduced that true Gaertner bacilli may be met with in the intestinal contents of rats and mice, a matter of importance in view of the frequent contamination of food by these animals.

Heuser (1910) examined 100 mice and in five isolated Gaertner bacilli of both types, i.e. *B. enteritidis* and *B. paratyphosus B* (*vel B. suipestifer* according to German classification), from their intestinal contents. The mice showed no symptoms of disease. He also examined about sixty white rats and found *B. enteritidis* but no *B. suipestifer*. He found that by animal passage bacilli of the *B. suipestifer* group showed a rise of virulence to rats.

Uhlenhuth (1909) examined twenty-five healthy mice and failed to find any Gaertner group organisms in the intestines or internal organs.

Zwick and Weichel (1911) examined 177 mice and in twenty-eight found Gaertner group bacilli present.

There is further evidence as to the occurrence of true Gaertner group bacilli in the intestines of rats and mice from certain feeding experiments. Mühlens, Darm and Fürst (1908) fed mice with different kinds of prepared food and a number of them died, Gaertner group bacilli being isolated. Gaertner group bacilli were not found in the foods by cultural tests. Zwick and Weichel fed 140 white mice with seventy samples of salt meat and different forms of pig, all of which culturally examined failed to show Gaertner group bacilli. Eighty-five (60·7 per cent.) of the mice died, and from two of them *B. paratyphosus B* was isolated.

These feeding experiments suggest that the Gaertner bacilli were present in the mice, probably in the intestines, and under the conditions of the experiments invaded the body and caused a general infection with death.

Savage and Read (1913) examined the internal organs and intestinal contents of forty-one rats. No Gaertner group bacilli were isolated from the intestinal contents, but five strains of *B. enteritidis* were obtained from the spleens (in two cases also from the liver) of different rats. In two instances Danysz's virus (*B. enteritidis*) had been distributed quite recently, while two and a half years previously the refuse tips and slaughter-houses from which these rats were obtained had been extensively dosed with this virus. It is highly probable that the bacilli isolated were derived (except in the two cases of recent infection) from an old infection with this virus, a conclusion supported by the failure to find this organism in the intestinal contents and by the fact that the serum from a number of these rats agglutinated *B. enteritidis* in high dilution.

A later investigation by the writer (Savage, 1918) confirms this hypothesis, since forty-eight rats obtained from a different source showed no Gaertner group bacilli or Gaertner group agglutinins.

It has already been recorded that rats and mice suffer from epidemics of disease due to this group of bacilli. In such outbreaks while many of the animals die a considerable percentage recover or even show few or no symptoms as a result of the infection. A consideration of the above investigations strongly suggests that these bacilli are not natural inhabitants of either rats or mice and that when found they occur in animals which have recovered from infection and are acting as carriers.

Petrie and O'Brien (1910) succeeded in experimentally producing the carrier-state in guinea-pigs by feeding them with *B. suipestifer*. In the case of two animals (out of six fed) the bacilli were isolated from the faeces for as long as fifty-nine days after the last feeding. The authors do not state if the bacillus used was virulent by injection when used for feeding, or if any impairment of virulence resulted from the sojourn in the alimentary tract of the guinea-pigs.

In an epizootic amongst the stock guinea-pigs at the Lister Institute due to *B. suipestifer*, recorded by O'Brien (1910), the survivors showed definite immunity to this bacillus, and five of them proved to be carriers, excreting the bacillus intermittently five months later.

Bainbridge (1912), in the Milroy Lectures for 1912, drew attention to the importance of the rat in relation to meat-poisoning, and suggested that the rat's intestine may be the true home of *B. enteritidis*, and that it reaches the alimentary canal of cattle and other domestic animals through the contamination of their food or bedding by rats.

C. In meat, particularly prepared meat.

In 1908 the writer (Savage, 1909) examined sixty-four specimens of brawn, sausage, tinned and other prepared foods, and also eighteen samples of pickling fluids from various sources. While pseudo- or para-Gaertner organisms were not uncommon, from only one sausage (out of twenty-eight) was a true Gaertner organism isolated. This was *B. enteritidis* and not *B. suipestifer*, although the sausage was a pork one. The particular sausage from which it was isolated was obtained from a small local butcher who made his sausages on the premises. No illness was known to result from consumption of the rest of the sausages.

On the whole the German investigations, which have been fairly numerous since 1908, are in accord with and confirm these results, but several workers have found the bacilli more frequently.

Mühlens, Darm and Fürst (1908) examined fifty-seven samples of different kinds of prepared meats bought in Berlin shops, and including pickled goose-breast, raw ham, cooked ham, smoked ham, smoked tongues, etc. In no case could they find any Gaertner group bacilli by cultural examination. When they fed white mice with the different foods, a large number of the mice died, and Gaertner group bacilli were isolated. Since, however, as already pointed out, mice feeding and inoculation methods are useless for this purpose (see also Reinhardt and Seibold, 1912 b, and Schellhorn, 1910), the essential value of their work is that they failed to find Gaertner group bacilli in these prepared foods by cultural examination.

Hübener (1908) examined 100 different varieties of sausage and isolated six Gaertner group bacilli, two from fresh blood sausages and four from smoked sausages. The cultural characters of the bacilli are not given.

Rimpau (1908) records that he found B. paratyphosus B in a liver sausage quite free from objectionable appearance or odour, and the use of which was in no way harmful.

Rommeler (1909) examined fifty-one samples of sausage, and in eight found paratyphoid bacilli, while from eight samples of "hackfleisch" in five he isolated the same bacillus. As no cultural, agglutination or inoculative experiments are given, it is not possible to say if he differentiated the true from the para-Gaertner forms.

Trautmann examined fifty-one samples of sausage, ham, goose-breast and smoked meat without finding any Gaertner group bacilli.

Zwick and Weichel (1910) culturally examined seventy samples of salt meat, goose-breast and different forms of prepared pig meat, and were unable to find any Gaertner bacilli.

Aumann investigated 150 specimens of sausage from Hamburg shops and failed to find Gaertner group bacilli in any of them.

Zweifel (1911) at Leipzig examined 248 specimens of chopped meat (hackfleisch), obtained quite fresh, both by direct plating and by enrichment method. In no case did he find true Gaertner group bacilli.

Ciurea (1912) working in Ostertag's laboratory examined fifty-three samples of "hackfleisch" from different Berlin sources. Although allied bacilli were isolated, in no instance was a true Gaertner group organism isolated.

Carey (1916) examined thirty-four samples of pork sausage at Chicago but no Gaertner group organisms were obtained from any of them.

These results may be taken as showing that true Gaertner group bacilli are nearly always absent from prepared meat foods, but that very occasionally they are present.

CHAPTER VII

FOOD POISONING OF UNSPECIFIC BACTERIAL ORIGIN

IT has been shown in Chapter V that all, or almost all, the larger and widespread outbreaks of bacterial food poisoning, where modern reliable methods have been employed to investigate them, have been found to be due to one or other member of the Gaertner group of bacilli. Although this is now admitted it is still advanced that a certain proportion of these larger outbreaks have a different bacterial origin. The great majority of the instances of outbreaks and attacks of food poisoning limited to one or two persons or members of one family, and these are probably very numerous, have never been systematically investigated and we are not, therefore, in a position to dogmatise as to their causation. To account for this residuum of larger outbreaks and these numerous unexplained limited attacks several explanations may be advanced.

In the first place there is a strong probability that not a few of these slighter and more localized outbreaks are also due to Gaertner group bacilli if only investigations were made. For others definite specific bacilli not of this group may be the cause, such as *B. faecalis alkaligenes, B. prodigiosus*, or bacilli at present unrecognized.

Two views, still widely favoured at the present time, have been advanced by different writers and investigators to account for many cases and outbreaks and require careful consideration. These two views are:

(*a*) That the food poisoning attacks are due to general bacterial mass infection not necessarily specific in nature.

(*b*) That the attacks are due to the changes caused by the action of putrefactive bacilli, in other words that the symptoms are due to the ingestion of food in a state of incipient or developed putrefaction.

General bacterial mass infection as a cause of food poisoning.

Not commonly definitely expressed, but certainly frequently assumed, is the hypothesis that outbreaks of food poisoning are caused, not by infection of the food with some specific bacillus, but through massive infection of the food with faecal and other bacilli, the symptoms being due to the action of the toxic products of these bacilli. This view is frequently suggested or implied as the explanation of individual outbreaks. The possibility of such a method of action cannot be ignored and the wide acceptance of this theory demands its careful consideration.

In its favour is the fact that many of the cardinal symptoms of food poisoning, such as diarrhoea, vomiting and some constitutional disturbance, are conditions which may be set up by any agencies which can disturb the balance of the alimentary tract. Amongst such agencies are certain chemical substances and it may well be that the toxic products of bacteria, such as *B. coli*, which in general possess low toxicity, may exert an irritant action sufficient to cause the symptoms of this condition.

A supposed analogy between food poisoning and epidemic diarrhoea has been utilised in this connection. Although the etiological view of epidemic diarrhoea most in vogue at the present time favours one or more specific bacteria as the cause, there is a considerable body of opinion which takes the view that the manifestations of epidemic diarrhoea in infants are nothing more than the result of massive bacterial infection, non-specific in nature, acting upon the sensitive mucous membrane of the infant. Delépine, for example, voiced this opinion in 1903 (Delépine, 1903), stating, "Epidemic diarrhoea of the common type occurring in this country is apparently in the great majority of instances the result of infection of food by bacilli belonging to the colon group of bacilli which are present at times in faecal matter. It appears that this infection of food does not generally lead to serious consequences unless the infection is massive from the first, or the food is kept for a sufficient length of time

and under conditions of temperature favouring the multiplication of these bacilli." His view at that time was that
"epidemic diarrhoea is generally the result of a more widely
disseminated, and less massive form of bacterial infection of
food than is the case with regard to the more definite outbreaks of food poisoning."

Consideration of the general facts and a study of detailed
outbreaks show almost insuperable difficulties in the way of
accepting this theory.

In the first place massive bacterial infection with intestinal
bacteria is exceedingly common and foods such as milk, ice-
cream, brawn and sausages are habitually consumed containing thousands of bacteria per cubic centimetre or
gramme, many of which are of direct intestinal origin.
Food poisoning outbreaks should be of repeated and constant
occurrence instead of being comparatively infrequent.

Further, there should be a *special* incidence upon the types
of food which are so frequently ingested loaded with excretal
bacteria. Milk in particular should be always causing outbreaks, yet if Chapter V is consulted it will be noted that
comparatively few outbreaks of definite food poisoning have
been traced to milk, and nearly all were due to bacterial
infection with a specific bacillus.

If outbreaks are caused by massive non-specific bacterial
infection we would expect to get a definite relationship
between dosage and the degree of infection. Those who ate
little would have slight symptoms, those who ate "not wisely
but too well" would pay the heavier price, the children with
their greater intestinal susceptibility would particularly be
selected. There would also be, in the more widespread outbreaks, a tailing off of the severity of the symptoms where
the infection was less massive. Nothing of this is the case,
the relationship between dose and severity of attack is at
most very inconstant and frequently non-existent, while
there is no special incidence on children.

In food poisoning outbreaks it is true that examination of
the food usually discloses faecal contamination, but it is
exceptional to find it different in kind or more massive in
character than food of similar nature, eaten without the

production of symptoms by thousands of other persons of the same age, sex and susceptibility.

A study of outbreaks, whether large or small, show that they are explosive in character, a characteristic especially associated with *specific* bacterial infection.

We have finally the impressive fact that the more carefully and fully individual outbreaks are studied and bacteriologically investigated the greater the number found to be associated with infection with some definite bacillus, and it is a reasonable assumption that the residuum of outbreaks unassociated in this way would be comparatively small if all were fully investigated, bacteriologically and chemically, and especially if material was available for examination early in the course of the outbreak.

This statement is substantiated by the occasional, almost chance, investigation of small outbreaks which differ in no way from others ascribed to massive bacterial infection, except that they happen to be investigated by competent bacteriologists. The following may be mentioned as an example:

In a small town a family consisting of a mother and her five children, aged four to twelve, consumed without harm their Sunday dinner of beefsteak pudding, greens and haricot beans, but all, except the mother, were taken ill, with the usual food poisoning symptoms, after consuming the remains of the beefsteak pudding for Monday's dinner. One of the children died. At the inquest the usual medical evidence as to ptomaine poisoning was given and the usual suggestions of bacterial multiplication and fermentation were advanced and no efforts were made to trace the source of infection, this hypothesis being accepted as a satisfactory explanation of everything. None of the food was submitted for bacteriological examination, nor were the internal organs of the fatal case bacteriologically investigated. The writer only became aware of the outbreak when it was too late to obtain such material but it was possible to obtain samples of blood from four of the children. These all showed the presence of agglutinins in marked amount for *B. enteritidis*, one of the food poisoning bacteria, thus conclusively demonstrating that this little outbreak was due to specific infection with this organism.

On the experimental side there is no evidence to support this hypothesis. Food very massively infected with *B. coli* and other intestinal bacteria given to animals to *eat* does not cause infection or illness, and there are no actual food poisoning outbreaks for which proof worth the name has been forthcoming that faecal *B. coli* have set up the condition. The only instance which the writer can trace showing that massive doses of *B. coli* taken into the human body by natural channels has caused symptoms is one recorded by Vaughan (1913). The Vaughans worked with large masses of *B. coli* grown for two weeks in agar in metal tanks. At the end of that time the crude bacterial substance obtained by extracting this mass with absolute alcohol and ether was powdered finely in an agate mortar for certain special investigations. They state "the person who did the pulverizing was often quite seriously poisoned during the process unless he took the precaution of wearing a mask which hindered the inhalation of the powder." Apart from symptoms due to direct irritation on the mucous membrane the chief symptoms were a feeling of depression and malaise and a chilly sensation. Occasionally a decided chill would be experienced, but no temperature readings were taken. Nausea and even vomiting were occasionally noted. After a period of discomfort varying from six to ten hours, during which the patient often complained of dull pains in the various joints, recovery would rapidly and completely take place.

In this case the dose of bacillus endotoxins was enormous, and it is significant that the symptoms are not those associated with food poisoning.

The question of the activities of *B. coli* as a putrefying organism is considered in the next section.

The view of the writer is that there is no evidence in favour of the hypothesis that ordinary massive bacterial food infection is a cause of food poisoning outbreaks. At the same time no one can make a close study of such outbreaks without coming across cases in which neither Gaertner group bacilli, *B. botulinus*, nor other recognized specific bacilli can be found and in which the possibility of putrefactive changes can be ruled out. In most such cases, however, opportunities for a *full* investigation have been lacking. The following will serve as an example of such an outbreak.

Six persons were taken ill after eating, on December 24th, 1917, of a dinner of which goose was the chief item, nine in all partaking of it. The symptoms included headache, giddiness, vomiting and a very irritating nettle rash. One of those who suffered ate no goose but had gravy and stuffing. It was stated, after the outbreak, that the goose smelt peculiarly whilst being cooked, also that there was a general complaint of the stuffing of sage and onions being bitter. The writer examined bacteriologically the carcase of the goose, but not until ten days after the dinner on December 24th, while none of the stuffing was obtainable. Comparatively few bacteria, aerobic or anaerobic, were present, *B. coli* being exceptionally scanty, while no Gaertner group bacilli were found. Examination of the blood of a number of the cases also helped to exclude infection with the latter group, and the cause of the outbreak had to be left unascertained. There was no evidence of putrefactive changes and the outbreak occurred during a very cold spell which with the bacteriological findings effectively disposed of the question of massive bacterial infection. The outbreak might have been due to chemical poisoning or to specific infection from some undetected anaerobic bacilli, and it will be noted that proper material was not available for a complete investigation.

The true causes of outbreaks of this nature can only be ascertained when complete and early investigations are possible and it is very desirable that opportunities for such examinations should be more frequently given and utilized.

Putrefactive bacilli and putrefactive changes as a cause of food poisoning.

It has been shown in Chapter I that the view that putrefactive changes are the cause of most outbreaks of food poisoning early obtained wide credence, and that the discovery of bodies of high toxicity to animals obtained from putrefying organic matter was hailed as giving the necessary basis of scientific support for this contention. The views so propounded were widely accepted as correct, and have obtained such a hold on both medical and lay opinion that even at the present time food poisoning outbreaks are promptly labelled as outbreaks of ptomaine poisoning by both the majority of medical men and the general public.

As a source of widespread outbreaks putrefactive changes can certainly be excluded, but, apart from these, expert opinion still favours the view that individual cases and limited outbreaks may be due to the consumption of meat in a state of early decomposition.

This view is also the basis of administrative action and enormous quantities of food in an early stage of putrefaction are seized and condemned as unfit. On grounds apart from any risk of causing food poisoning outbreaks strong justification may be advanced for such action, but at the same time it is highly desirable that administrative procedure on so extensive a scale should rest on a firm basis of scientifically ascertained fact and not on any supposed harmfulness due to ptomaines which, as will be shown later, is devoid of scientific foundation or on unsubstantiated statements repeated and copied from textbook to textbook without any effort to analyse and verify.

It is therefore of material importance to consider in some detail the bacteriological and chemical changes which are included under the term "putrefaction" and the evidence pointing to the potential harmfulness to man of the consumption of food in such a condition.

The chemical changes which take place in putrefaction.

By putrefaction is understood the decomposition of organic matter, chiefly protein in character, by the action of bacteria, by which it is split up into a number of chemical substances many of which are gaseous and foul smelling. Earlier observers considered putrefaction to be a kind of fermentation similar, for example, to the production of alcohol from sugar, and it was left to Pasteur to show that bacteria were the cause.

The decomposition changes in non-nitrogenous matter are hardly of the nature of putrefaction so that for practical purposes consideration may be confined to changes in the proteins.

To understand clearly the degradation changes in proteins as a result of putrefaction it is necessary to give a brief account of the composition of the animal proteins and their simpler cleavage products.

The proteins are highly complex compounds of C, H, O, N and S, belonging for the most part to the colloids. The protein molecule is a very large one. Some fifty or so natural proteins are known, occurring in both animals and plants, and they are classified according to their origin, solubility in solvents such as water, saline solutions and alcohol, coagulability on heating and other physical characters.

The work of Emil Fischer and his pupils has confirmed and elaborated the theory originally propounded by Hofmeister, that the protein molecule is built up of a series of amino-acids[1] forming a class of products which have been designated the polypeptides by Fischer. Such polypeptides form the essential part of the structure of the protein molecule, but it may contain other groups, such as phosphoric acid and possibly also carbohydrates.

Under the influence of chemical agencies, such as acids or

---

[1] The amino-acids are bodies in which a NH_2 group (the amino group) is substituted for a hydrogen atom of the carbon group nearest the acid radical. For example, acetic acid is a simple fatty acid with the formula CH_3—COOH, while CH_2NH_2—COOH is amino-acetic acid or glycocoll. The aromatic amino-acids are those in which amino-acids are united to the benzene ring. Tyrosine belongs to this group. The general formula of the mono-amido acids may be stated as $R—CH{\Large<}^{NH_2}_{COOH}$ where R may be of very simple or very complicated structure; for example, simple chains as in leucine, members of the aromatic series as in tyrosine or tryptophane or sulphur containing bodies.

In the di-amino acids two hydrogen atoms are replaced by NH_2 groups and these have the general formula $R—C{\Large<}^{NH_2}_{COOH}$ with NH_2. Lysine, histidine and cystine belong to this group.

alkalies, physical agencies such as superheated steam, the action of digestive or other ferments or the activities of bacteria, the protein molecule is decomposed and various cleavage products form. These substances may be classed as primary cleavage products, i.e. those which exist as radicals within the molecule, or as secondary products, i.e. those not existing pre-formed in the molecule but formed by transformation of the primary products.

"When the protein molecule is broken down in the laboratory by processes similar to those brought about by the digestive enzymes which occur in the alimentary canal, the essential change is due to what is called *hydrolysis*: that is, the molecule unites with the water and then breaks up into smaller molecules. The first cleavage products, which are called *proteoses*, retain many of the characters of the original protein; and the same is true, though to a less degree, of the *peptones*, which come next in order of formation. The peptones in their turn are decomposed into short linkages of amino-acids which are called *polypeptides*, and finally the individual amino-acids are obtained separated from each other" (Halliburton, 1916).

It is important to realize that whatever method is used to decompose the protein molecule the process goes through all these stages and approximately quantitatively as well as qualitatively. Different agencies however carry the process to different stages and the characteristic chemical products brought about by putrefactive bacteria are due to their carrying the processes further and causing extensive secondary cleavage changes.

The conversions into proteoses, peptones and amino-acids are therefore changes which are common to all methods by which the protein molecule is dissociated, and chief interest centres upon the further changes in the amino-acids brought about by the putrefactive bacteria. Bacteria (and other fungi) are peculiar in being able to break down the amino-acids into bases and acids which, in general, have not been demonstrated as products of the metabolism of animals and the higher plants.

As long ago as 1902 Czapek, and also Emmerling, pointed

out that the amino-acids furnish bacteria with abundant and available nutritive material. The amino-acids are non-toxic bodies and include substances such as glycine (amino-acetic acid), alanine (amino-propionic acid), leucine (iso-butyl-α-amino-acetic acid), tyrosine, cystine, aspartic acid, glutamic acid, histidine and tryptophane.

The secondary degradation products which result include bodies such as indol, skatol, skatol-carboxylic acid, skatol-acetic acid, phenyl propionic acid, phenyl acetic acid, p-cresol and phenol. In addition a number of simple bodies, such as ammonia, methane, carbon dioxide, sulphuretted hydrogen, hydrogen, etc., are formed as end-products.

The precise chemical bodies which will be formed will depend upon a number of factors, such as the character of the bacteria concerned, the conditions of growth (especially as regards the presence or absence of oxygen), the available sources of nutriment other than the amino-acids, the temperature and the stage of the process.

Hopkins and Cole (1903), for example, studied the changes produced in chemically pure tryptophane by putrefaction. They obtained indol, skatol, and skatol-carbonic acid by the action of aerobic bacteria and skatol-acetic acid with anaerobic organisms, in this way showing that the tryptophane radical is the precursor of these substances in putrefaction.

In the same way tyrosine is the precursor of phenol, para-cresol, para-oxy-phenyl acetic acid and other bodies.

Most, if not all, of the sulphur in the protein molecule is contained in the amino-acid cystine and the offensive sulphur-containing bodies, such as hydrogen sulphide, methyl mercaptan (CH_3SH) and ethyl mercaptan, produced during putrefaction are due to the breaking down of this amino-acid.

In addition to these numerous products a very definite group of bodies, chemically of the nature of amines, are formed in the later stages of putrefaction, and to these bodies, owing to the high toxicity possessed by some of them, the very greatest importance has been attached as a cause of bacterial food poisoning.

A very characteristic action of putrefactive bacteria generally is their power to split off carbon dioxide from the carboxyl (COOH) group of the amino-acids with the production of amines according to the following equation:

$$NH_2-R-COOH = NH_2-R-H + CO_2.$$

In this way a whole series of bodies is formed which include the ptomaines of Selmi and Brieger and other bases, some of which are capable of exerting a poisonous action on man and animals. This decarboxylation of amino-acids seems to be a general reaction of a good many putrefactive organisms.

As examples of such changes it may be mentioned that di-amino-valeric acid is converted into putrescine, di-amino-caproic acid (lysine) into cadaverine, and tyrosine into tyramine. In the same way the poisonous and probably important body β-imidazolethylamine is the amine of histidine. The decarboxylation of amino-acids is not necessarily accompanied by a putrefactive odour or other obvious sign of bacterial action, but as Barger points out in the absence of bacteria decarboxylation of amino-acids does not occur.

It is important to remember that ptomaines, in sharp contradistinction to toxins, are non-specific, i.e. they are not the products of intracellular metabolism specifically characteristic of the organisms which produce them. They are merely degradation products of the protein molecule and are elaborated by all bacteria that are capable of producing this degree of protein cleavage when grown on a suitable nutrient medium and under favourable conditions of growth. They may be produced by bacteria which possess no pathogenic power, while on the other hand highly pathogenic bacteria which are not powerful protein splitting organisms may produce little or no ptomaines.

Owing to the importance which is still attached by some writers to these bodies and their historical interest, particulars of a few are given. For an extended account see Vaughan and Novy's book, *Cellular Toxins* (1903).

Methylamine, CH_3NH_2. This is the simplest amine and has been obtained from decomposing herring, haddock and other fish. It does not possess any toxic action and very similar remarks apply to di- and tri-methylamine and to ethylamine.

Putrescine (tetramethylenediamine) has been obtained from putrefying fish and other organic matter. Although recognizable about the fourth day of putrefaction it does not occur in appreciable quantity until about the eleventh day, while the amount increases as putrefaction continues.

Cadaverine is similar in composition to putrescine with the addition of another CH_2 group. It has been isolated from the putrefaction products of many forms of protein. It can also be obtained from the amino-acid lysine by bacterial action.

Van Slyke and Hart (1903) found a little putrescine in ordinary Cheddar cheese. Once formed putrescine and cadaverine appear to be very resistant to bacterial action.

Putrescine and cadaverine are of interest because they have been found in the intestine, derived from the putre-factive decomposition of proteins, and sometimes in the urine in cystinuria. They are said to have some physio-logical properties, setting up, according to Behring, poisonous symptoms in mice, rabbits and guinea-pigs. Udránszky and Beauman, however, failed to obtain any evidence of intes-tinal irritation when dogs were fed with enormous doses of cadaverine.

The choline group of ptomaines includes choline, neurine, muscarine and betaine and is of more interest.

Choline is a normal constituent of every cell, forming the nitrogenous portion of the lecithin molecule. It is only very moderately toxic, but the closely related neurine into which it may be transformed is highly poisonous. It has been suggested that one form of food intoxication is due to the choline, obtained from the lecithin in the food, being con-verted in the gastro-intestinal tract into neurine.

Brieger obtained neurine in the putrefaction products of horse, beef and human blood after five to six days action in summer.

Muscarine was obtained, accompanied by choline, by Schmiedeberg and Koppe from poisonous mushrooms.

Both neurine and muscarine are extremely poisonous and very similar in their action. Subcutaneous injection of but 1 to 3 mg. of muscarine in man produces salivation, rapid pulse, reddening of the face, weakness, depression, profuse sweating, vomiting and diarrhoea. Neurine acts very similarly. "The toxicity of these substances is so great that not a large amount would need to be formed by oxidation of choline to produce severe symptoms, although it is not known that this occurs actually in the body. When introduced by the mouth, the lethal dose of neurine is ten times as great as when injected subcutaneously, indicating that chemical changes in the gastro-intestinal tract offer some protection against intoxication by these substances when taken in tainted food. Choline, although by no means so poisonous as neurine, has a similar action when administered in sufficiently large doses. According to Brieger it is about $\frac{1}{10}$ to $\frac{1}{20}$ as toxic as neurine" (Wells, *Chemical Pathology*).

Mytilotoxine is chiefly of interest in that it is said to be the specific poison in connection with mussel poisoning and was obtained by Brieger in 1885 from toxic mussels. He was, however, unable to obtain it from ordinary mussels which were allowed to putrefy for sixteen days. According to Brieger it produces all the characteristic effects seen in mussel poisoning. Its connection with mussel poisoning is considered on p. 132.

Alimentary toxaemia.

Before considering the bacteriology of putrefaction or the part ptomaines or other putrefactive products play in food poisoning it is desirable, as throwing some light upon the problem, to briefly discuss some facts which have been elicited in connection with the question of alimentary toxaemia in the human subject. This is a matter upon which great differences of opinion are encountered and indeed is one which bristles with difficulties. It bears upon the question of putrefaction since it is evident that processes closely analogous to putrefaction take place in the intestine of animals, not only abnormally but normally, with the production of very similar products.

It has already been pointed out that the primary degradation products of protein decomposition are the same whether caused by putrefactive bacteria or by the action of enzymes in ordinary digestion. According to Strasburger at least one

third of the faeces in man consists of bacteria, while in
diarrhoea this proportion is even greatly increased. Indol,
skatol, phenol, and cresol are all bodies which are formed in
the alimentary tract by bacterial action upon the proteins
and when formed in excess they are absorbed by the intestines, oxidized into indoxyl, skatoxyl, etc., and eliminated
in the urine.

The toxic effects of indol and skatol are not very striking
when given by the mouth, but symptoms such as irritability,
headache and flight of ideas are recorded by Herter (1907)
after feeding with large doses of indol. He notes that the
quantity of indol administered to produce these symptoms
was probably in excess of any amount that would be absorbed from the intestine, even in the most pronounced
pathological condition.

It has been suggested that the indol in the intestine may
be, in part at least, a product of ordinary intracellular
protein metabolism, but the experiments of Ellinger and
Gentzen (1903) showed that tryptophane when fed or injected subcutaneously causes no increase in indican in the
urine, whereas its injection into the caecum causes much
indicanuria thus demonstrating that it results only from
intestinal putrefaction.

The formation of amines, identical with or allied to the
ptomaines of Brieger, has also been demonstrated in the
human intestine. As already mentioned the di-amines
putrescine and cadaverine have been found in the urine and
faeces in cases of cystinuria, while they have also been found
in the stools of cholera patients; further, cadaverine has
been found by Dombrowski in the faeces of a healthy man.
In view, however, of their low toxicity they can hardly be
regarded as likely sources of toxaemia to any serious extent.

In recent years a number of interesting examples have been
brought forward showing that in the intestine certain of the
non-toxic amino-acids may be converted into poisonous
amines by decarboxylation through bacterial action. Tyrosine under the action of faecal bacilli has been converted into
tyramine by Barger and Walpole, while by the same agencies
tryptophane is converted into its corresponding poisonous

amine. Tyramine has indeed been found to occur in ripened cheese due to bacterial action upon the tyrosine in the cheese.

Of special interest is the base β-imidazolethylamine (or β-i) produced from histidine by splitting off carbon dioxide. It was first prepared synthetically by Windham and Vogt (1907), and then by Ackermann (1910), who obtained it by the action of putrefactive bacteria on histidine. About the same time it was detected in ergot and its physiological action investigated by Dale and Laidlaw. Mellanby and Twort demonstrated that it was produced in the alimentary canal and isolated a bacillus of the colon type from the intestines capable of producing it from histidine, while Berthelot has also isolated a bacillus from the intestine with this property. It is important to note that Mellanby and Twort found their bacillus as an inhabitant of the normal intestine and not in abnormal conditions only such as epidemic diarrhoea.

Summarising available facts it would appear to be established that bodies possessing poisonous properties, indol, skatol, and especially certain poisonous amines, are produced from the cleavage of proteins by bacterial action in the *normal* intestine. It is further evident that under ordinary circumstances the human organism is capable of dealing with them without the production of any symptoms. This defensive mechanism has not been fully explained, but as long ago as 1899 Herter and Wakeman showed that the living cells of the body, especially the hepatic and renal cells and the epithelial cells of the intestinal tract, have the power of absorbing considerable quantities of indol as well as of phenol and combining with them so that these bodies cannot be recovered by distillation. The discrepancy between the fatal dose of toxins given by the mouth compared with when introduced under the skin is usually very great and postulates a powerful defensive mechanism. The liver would appear to have very marked powers of destroying both toxins and alkaloids.

The facts considered under alimentary toxaemia show that it is not sufficient to demonstrate that the food (putrefactive or otherwise) contains chemical bodies which exhibit toxic properties when introduced into the body under maximal favourable circumstances. To cause symptoms we have in addition to postulate some breaking down of the defensive mechanism, possibly in the first place of the mucous membrane of the intestine, allowing their absorption and non-destruction by the liver.

The bacteriology of putrefaction.

Although a good deal of work has been done on the subject of putrefaction the bulk of it is chemical in nature and the bacteriological studies usually refer only to the activities of certain selected organisms. Undoubtedly the chemical changes which make up the process of putrefaction can be brought about by many bacteria, while in ordinary putre-faction it seems fairly certain that we have to deal with the activities of both aerobic and anaerobic bacteria.

Putrefactive anaerobes.

There are really two separate points to consider: the known anaerobes which possess putrefactive properties and the anaerobes actually concerned in putrefaction as met with under natural conditions.

As regards the latter point the subject has not been ade-quately studied, and we are not in a position to define the chief anaerobes taking part in natural putrefaction or even to affirm that there are any anaerobes which are so invari-ably present in putrefactive material and which take such a conspicuous part in the processes of putrefaction as to be fairly given the title of "putrefactive" anaerobes. Many of the organisms described below have been isolated from putrescent matter, but our knowledge of the relative import-ance and activities of the different types is still very indefinite. The classification of anaerobes is decidedly unsatisfactory, but considerable progress has been made recently, chiefly in connection with the investigation of these organisms in war wounds.

Putrefaction being essentially a degradation of the protein molecule the activities of anaerobes in this direction must largely turn upon their biochemical characters, and from this point of view Rettger (1908) has grouped them into four classes.

(a) Those that produce very little or no putrefactive change or fermentation. B. *tetani* is a good example.

(b) Those with a strong putrefactive action on natural proteins but which fail in fermentative properties, as illustrated by B. *putrificus*.

(c) Those which are primarily fermentative organisms and whose putrefactive functions are very slight or perhaps absent. For example, B. *welchii*.

(d) Those which have very marked putrefactive and fermentative properties, as shown best in the bacillus of malignant oedema and the bacillus of symptomatic anthrax.

A simpler classification is that given by McIntosh (1917) into non-proteolytic and proteolytic anaerobes.

Of anaerobes possessing well-marked putrefactive properties the following may be mentioned:

B. *putrificus*. First described by Bienstock (1884), who found it in great abundance in ordinary street dust. The same bacillus was isolated by Klein from putrefying dead bodies and called by him B. *cadaveris sporogenes*. Bienstock also found his bacillus widely distributed in faeces and putrefying material but never in the faeces of normal individuals. Passini and also Rettger however state that this organism does occur in normal faeces, but there is some doubt as to the identity of their bacilli with the true B. *putrificus*. Although widespread in nature it is difficult to isolate. A long slender bacillus which produces large terminal spores and then closely resembles B. *tetani*. Actively motile and Gram positive. Cultures have a strong putrid odour. According to McIntosh it ferments glucose, maltose, lactose, saccharose and starch, clots milk, frequently with partial digestion, and liquefies coagulated serum in two to three days. It is non-pathogenic to guinea-pigs by subcutaneous or intraperitoneal injection.

Vibrion septique or Bacillus of malignant oedema. Until recently the descriptions of this organism have been indefinite and variable and undoubtedly different bacteria have been included under this title. This organism is usually isolated from infected animals, is common in wounds and is said to occur in soil and putrefactive material and to be a constant inhabitant of the normal intestinal tract (Mace and others). The latter point is doubtful.

A good account of its cultural characters is given by Robertson (1918) of which the following points are of interest in the present connection. A saccharolytic organism clotting milk in three to seven days, without putrefactive or digestive reaction on meat and inspissated serum. Spores are readily formed upon all media; they are oval in shape and central or subterminal in position. The organism is pathogenic for man and also for laboratory animals, producing a blood-stained oedema and deep red colour of the infected muscles.

B. sporogenes. A widespread organism common in animal excreta and cultivated soil. A large motile bacillus sporing readily, the spores being usually subterminal. It digests milk and liquefies coagulated serum and also possesses some saccharolytic properties, fermenting glucose and maltose. In albumin containing media it produces an unpleasant putrid smell. Grown on meat it blackens it. It is non-pathogenic.

B. welchii. Under this title is included a group of organisms with very strong fermentative but trifling proteolytic pro-perties. *B. perfringens* of Veillon and Zuber, *B. aerogenes capsulatus* and *B. enteritidis sporogenes* of Klein (a mixture) are all names of organisms identical with one or other types of this bacillus. These bacilli have been described as putre-factive organisms by Tissier (1912) and others, but they do not liquefy coagulated serum, peptonise milk or produce a putrefactive odour. Pathogenic to laboratory animals.

For a good description of these and other anaerobes McIntosh's (1917) Report may be consulted. They are men-tioned here as organisms commonly associated with putre-faction, but as stated above their exact activities in this direction are very doubtful. While several are pathogenic by injection none are known to be hurtful when given by the mouth. Indeed the spores of several of them are natural inhabitants of animal excreta, as indeed is the very patho-genic *B. tetani.* Metchnikoff fed dogs with huge quantities of *B. perfringens* (*B. welchii*), such as 200 to 500 c.c. of broth cultures, and noted progressive loss of weight with slight anaemia and, when the animals were killed, some evidence of sclerotic changes in the kidneys. As Ledingham (1913) remarks it is surprising that nothing worse happened after such heroic dosing.

Putrefactive aerobes.

Those to which the greatest share in putrefactive changes have been ascribed are the proteus family (particularly *Proteus vulgaris*) and to a lesser extent *B. coli* and allied bacteria. It is probable that many sporing aerobes, such as *B. subtilis* and its allies, also play a part in putrefaction.

The putrefactive properties of *B. proteus* (using the term as a convenient general one to cover *Proteus vulgaris* and other strains of this family) seem to have been a good deal exaggerated. According to most observers these organisms can invariably be isolated from putrid meat (see Addendum IV), but this is not the writer's experience as regards *Proteus vulgaris*.

All the members of this family are short, actively motile, Gram negative, non-sporing bacilli, aerobic and grow better at 20–25° C. than at 37° C. Their characteristic gelatine colonies are well known and the gelatine is rapidly liquefied. Cultures in materials containing albumin or gelatine have a putrefactive odour and become alkaline. They produce indol, ferment glucose, saccharose and maltose but not lactose. Milk is clotted and then peptonized. Coagulated serum is liquefied.

While the above gives the characteristic characters of a typical strain of *B. proteus* there are many variations and the group is a very ill-defined one.

Rettger and Newell (1912) tested a large number of *B. proteus* strains and found that they had no power to initiate changes in proteins. When other sources of nitrogen (peptones, etc.) are present, however, this organism will rapidly attack proteins. Herter and Broeck (1911), for example, remark from their work, "The study of the products of the growth of Proteus shows that, to some extent at least, it is a putrefactive organism. It destroys a native albumin (casein) and it produces ammonia, primary amines, hydrogen sulphide, fatty acids of a high molecular weight, aromatic oxyacids, indol and indol acetic acids, all of which are associated with putrefaction."

Tissier (1912) found that the action of B. *proteus* upon albumin is qualitatively less (i.e. about two-thirds) than that of the putrefactive aerobes, but that B. *proteus* splits up the protein molecule much further. The products never give the biuret reaction, the quantity of amino-acids is always less and the quantity of ammonia always greater.

The putrefactive abilities of B. *coli* are said to be somewhat similar, but less marked than those of B. *proteus*.

No definite studies have been made of the large number of other aerobes which play a part in the putrefactive disintegration of the protein molecule. Scientific investigation on modern lines is very desirable.

The relative share of anaerobes and aerobes in putrefaction.

Pasteur considered that putrefaction could only occur in the absence of free oxygen, and this view was upheld by Nencki, Bienstock and other workers. In putrefaction, as it actually occurs, it is evident that both aerobes and anaerobes play a part but something depends upon the interpretation of the word "putrefaction." Thus Rettger (1908), using the term in the restricted sense of only including the bacterial decomposition of albuminous matter accompanied by the formation of foul smelling substances, takes the view that the action of the obligate aerobes is one of ordinary dissolution or digestion and that real putrefaction is the work of obligate anaerobes alone.

Bainbridge (1911) showed that certain anaerobic bacteria, including B. *coli*, B. *enteritidis*, B. *proteus*, *Staphylococcus pyogenes aureus*, were unable of themselves to attack and decompose pure egg-albumin and serum-protein. Sperry and Rettger (1915) confirmed these observations and also showed that certain putrefactive anaerobes (B. *putrificus*, B. *oedematis maligni*, B. *anthracis-symptomatici*) are also devoid of this property. The observations to the same effect of Rettger and Newell with proteus strains have already been mentioned.

Rettger, Berman and Sturges (1916) carried the work a stage further and showed that these organisms, aerobes and anaerobes alike, were unable to initiate decomposition changes in proteins when the latter were the only source of nitrogen. When soluble proteins (peptones and proteoses) were tested the non-gelatine liquefying organisms acted similarly, but the gelatine liquefiers such as *Staphylococcus aureus, Proteus vulgaris, B. subtilis* and *B. prodigiosus* rapidly decomposed the soluble proteins into products which no longer gave the biuret reaction. In other words the proteins were only attacked if a proteolytic enzyme was also present. If the cultural methods adopted were such that the bacilli added contained no enzymes, even the gelatine liquefiers could not decompose pure proteins.

The term "putrefaction" covers an exceedingly complex series of changes in organic matter of the highest chemical complexity. It is evident that under natural conditions, when numerous types of bacteria gain access to the decomposing material, many different organisms are given an opportunity to play a part. Bacteria, such as *B. subtilis*, which produce proteolytic ferments may be spoken of as putrefactive organisms equally with types such as *B. putrificus*, since they produce enzymes which alter proteins into bodies upon which the true putrefactive bacilli can act. We can adopt the narrow terminology of Rettger and exclude these organisms as non-putrefactive, but taking the broader view of putrefaction as embracing the whole range of the changes from the preliminary hydrolysis of the protein molecule to the production of foul smelling bodies it is obvious that aerobes and anaerobes both play a part in it, and it is not possible with present knowledge to accurately disentangle their several activities. Under certain circumstances on the other hand (for example, in tinned meats) changes comparable to if not identical with putrefactive changes may occur and be the work of one or two types of bacilli. More investigations in this direction are desirable.

Critical consideration of the evidence incriminating putrefactive food as a cause of food poisoning.

While tainted meat is nearly universally accepted as a cause of illness the facts already given show that no very clear evidence is available as to why precisely such food is harmful.

The possibilities of harm appear limited to one or more of the following:

1. Due to the toxic action of degradation products of the protein molecule.

2. Due to toxins (endo- or exo-) produced by the growth of definite putrefactive bacilli in the food outside the body.

3. Due to the ingestion of putrefactive bacilli which elaborate their poisons and exert their toxic action in the human intestine.

The first possibility is non-specific, the two latter suggest that certain of the putrefactive bacteria are specifically pathogenic.

Each may be considered in detail.

Due to toxic protein degradation products. It has been shown that the chemical changes grouped under the term putrefaction are brought about by the activities of many bacteria, both aerobes and anaerobes, and consist of the production of a large series of chemical substances formed out of, and due to the breaking down of, the protein molecule. These substances are not specific products produced exclusively by putrefactive bacilli, but are products common to all agencies which have the power to break down proteins.

The most striking of these bodies, since a number of them possess markedly poisonous properties, are the diamines isolated and studied by Brieger and others and known as ptomaines. Not unnaturally the demonstration of the production of such highly toxic bodies during putrefaction led to a wide acceptance of the view that these bodies were the cause not only of the harmfulness of tainted meat but of food poisoning in general, a view crystallized by the wide acceptance of the term "ptomaine poisoning" as one synonymous with food poisoning.

As regards ptomaines these bodies appear to be present in putrefying organic matter if the processes are allowed to go on long enough. These poisonous amines are not however produced in the early but only in the later stages of putrefaction and usually do not begin to appear until putrefaction has been in progress for a week. A study of the work of the earlier investigators, who isolated and determined their pathological properties, shows that they were only isolated by them after putrefaction had been allowed to continue under optimum conditions for some time, usually several weeks, and long after the most obtrusive signs of putrefaction had set in. They represent *late* protein degradation products. Under ordinary commercial conditions no one would be stupid enough to vend such food, no one would be rash enough to eat it. In other words, ptomaines are only produced when the food is far too nasty to eat.

In the second place the toxicity of ptomaines when administered by natural channels has been enormously exaggerated. The view of the intensely poisonous properties of ptomaines was almost entirely founded upon the results of *inoculation* experiments in animals. The introduction of such bodies alien to the animal economy direct into the tissues might very well set up toxic symptoms and there is a whole range of substances, such as snake venoms, products of pathogenic organisms, etc., which are nearly harmless by the mouth but intensely toxic when introduced under the skin. It is well known that many bacterial toxins, such as tetanus toxin, are extremely pathogenic by inoculation, but for which relatively enormous doses must be given by the mouth to induce any symptoms.

Experiments demonstrating toxicity by the mouth for these ptomaines are very few, and the writer has not come across any direct evidence that feeding with ptomaines prepared from putrefying meat has reproduced the symptoms of food poisoning.

It must also be mentioned that the methods by which ptomaines have been isolated are very faulty and the majority of the experiments have been undertaken with impure bodies, and some of the symptoms produced were

probably due to these impurities. Boeklish long ago showed
that in preparing ptomaines from putrefying fish the most
poisonous properties were possessed by the extraction fluid
freshly prepared from putrefying broth. During the process
of preparing the bases the toxicity of the extract diminished.
Klein fed some mice on portions of a meat pie which had given
rise to symptoms of poisoning in human beings and the mice
were made ill and died; after keeping the pie for a few days
it acquired an intense odour of putrefaction and at the same
time lost its poisonous properties; mice fed on it remained
unaffected.

Ptomaines being disposed of there yet remains the possibility that other non-specific protein degradation products
produced in putrefaction may cause food poisoning symptoms. It has already been explained that protein decomposition products identical with those produced in putrefaction are normally produced in the human intestine and
that, for the most part, they cause no symptoms or meta-
bolic disturbance. Some of these bodies, e.g. sulphuretted
hydrogen, indol and skatol, possess toxic properties, but only
when introduced into the body in some way other than by
the alimentary canal or when given in very large and continued doses. The writer has carried out several series of
experiments which show how late these bodies are produced
in the ordinary putrefaction of meat and it is evident that
they are not produced in sufficient quantities in decomposing meat at any stage at which enough would be eaten to
cause food poisoning attacks. Indeed the recorded symptoms
from the ingestion of large quantities of these substances are
not those associated with an outbreak of food poisoning.
When the subject of alimentary toxaemia was discussed it
was shown that the defensive powers of the animal organism
to protect itself from these non-specific protein degradation
products present in the intestine are very considerable and
effective. For any of these degradation products to be a
cause of food poisoning we must postulate their *early* appearance in the food in such quantities that they can upset the
protective mechanism of the body (intestinal cells, liver,
etc.) to such an extent that they will be absorbed in amounts

large enough to cause symptoms. It is a possible hypothesis, but not only does there happen to be no evidence to support it, but on the other hand the writer has found that these bodies are not produced in meat in any quantity at stages at which anyone would be likely to eat it.

Consideration of the above facts makes it most unlikely that the symptoms of food poisoning are due to any of the ordinary non-specific degradation products of the protein molecule, while as regards one group of them—the ptomaines —it must be accepted as certain that they play no part in food poisoning resulting from food putrefaction.

The term "ptomaine poisoning" is clearly incorrect and its retention is unfortunate and misleading as it leads to a faulty conception of the pathology of the condition, and what is worse to the neglect of proper methods of investigation and prevention. It is to be hoped that it will speedily be relegated to the limbo reserved for unsubstantiated theories.

Due to toxins produced by the activities of putrefactive bacilli. The important part taken by anaerobes in putrefaction has been explained and it is a feasible hypothesis that these and certain putrefactive aerobes might produce specific toxins (exo-toxins or endo-toxins). Apart from *B. botulinus*, which is not a putrefactive anaerobe, there is no evidence of the formation by these organisms of toxins which are pathogenic when introduced by the mouth. Some of the putrefactive anaerobes, such as *B. sporogenes* and *B. putrificus*, are quite non-pathogenic even by injection; other anaerobes, such as *B. welchii* or *Vibrion septique*, possess marked pathogenic properties when injected into laboratory animals, causing severe local and general symptoms and usually death. They also produce toxins which reproduce the symptoms on injection. These facts suggest that these toxin producing anaerobes might be responsible for poisonous properties in decomposing food, but this hypothesis is negatived by the fact that they are not toxic when fed and indeed several of them, including the powerful toxin producer *B. welchii*, are natural intestinal inhabitants.

As regards the putrefactive aerobes it is constantly stated

that *B. proteus* is a cause of food poisoning. This claim is based in part on the fact that it is a powerful protein decomposing organism, in part because it is an organism possessed of some toxicity and lastly because it has been found etiologically associated with a number of outbreaks of food poisoning.

The first part of the claim has been dealt with when the general toxicity of the protein degradation products was discussed. The pathogenicity of this group of organisms is discussed in detail in Addendum IV (p. 123). It is there shown that while they may cause toxic symptoms by injection the evidence is conflicting and weak as to their pathogenicity when introduced by feeding. Certain strains do exhibit toxic properties when fed, but there is no clear evidence that anything comparable to an attack of food poisoning can be induced.

The association of *B. proteus* with food poisoning outbreaks is discussed in Addendum V (p. 126). This shows that for most of the outbreaks reported as due to *B. proteus* the evidence is of the slenderest, while for none of them is definite proof forthcoming.

The writer has carried out a number of feeding experiments with putrid meat the details of which have not yet been published. For example five different kittens were fed with highly putrid meat from different sources, each animal receiving from three to six feeds, usually on consecutive days, with watery emulsions of the decomposed meat. No signs of food poisoning resulted while, apart from a considerable but often temporary loss of weight, or diminution of rate of natural increase, no symptoms were observable. In contrast with these a rabbit injected subcutaneously with but 1 c.c. of washings from three days' old putrid meat died four days after the injection. In this case no bacterial cause of death could be detected, but in another instance *B. welchii* was recovered from the tissues and the post-mortem appearances accorded with death from that organism.

These experiments support the contentions expressed as to the absence of toxins in putrid meat capable of causing symptoms by feeding.

Due to putrefactive bacilli elaborating poisonous toxins in the alimentary tract. This view suggests that the conditions in the intestinal tract are likely to be especially favourable for the elaboration of such toxins and is merely an extension of the view already dealt with. If these putrefactive bacilli cannot elaborate poisons *in vitro* it seems unlikely they can do so *in vivo* and there is no evidence. Also such a view requires some incubation period to allow of their formation, and in cases of putrid meat poisoning it is generally stated there is little or no incubation period.

Dealing with putrefaction generally and without attempting to restrict it to the activities of the products of *B. proteus* or any single bacillus, it may be said that available evidence is at present insufficient to establish that putrefactive changes are a cause of food poisoning. As a cause of extensive outbreaks putrefaction can certainly be excluded. Apart from these we are still left with a possibility that limited outbreaks and individual attacks of illness may be due to the consumption of meat in a state of early decomposition. In such cases the symptoms can conceivably be due to the protein degradation products which result from the chemical changes caused by putrefactive bacilli, whether amines or the products of further disintegration such as indol, skatol, mercaptan, etc., but to acquiesce in this hypothesis we must suppose that the quantities of such degradation products swept into the intestine when tainted food is consumed are so considerable in amount that the defensive mechanism of the body is for the time overborne, and either these poisonous bodies, or others naturally present in the intestine, are absorbed and reach the circulation in amounts capable of producing definite symptoms. While the possibility of such a succession of events cannot be altogether rejected there is no reliable evidence, that the writer has been able to unearth, that it does occur.

Another, and on the whole more probable, supposition is that the symptoms must be ascribed to specific toxins elaborated by certain of the putrefactive bacilli. At present, however, there is no reliable data associating any putrefactive bacillus with the production of such specific toxins acting through the intestinal tract, but it is possible that noxious effects might be exerted by the toxins of two or more acting symbiotically.

Tainted food is universally suspect, possibly quite justifiably suspect, but neither the degree of its malevolence nor the precise cause of its harmfulness has been placed upon a scientific foundation.

REFERENCES.

(Including Addenda IV and V.)

Ackermann (1910). *Zeit. f. physiol. Chemie*, LXV. 504.

Bainbridge (1911). *Journ. of Hygiene*, XI. 341.

Barger (1914). *The Simpler Natural Bases* (Monographs on Biochemistry).

Barger and Walpole (1909). *Journ. of Physiol.* XXXVIII. 343.

Berthelot (1913). *Compt. rend. de la Soc. de Biologie*, LXXIV. 575.

—— (1914 *a*). *Ann. de l'Inst. Pasteur*, XXVIII. 132.

—— (1914 *b*). *Ibid.* XXVIII. 839, 913.

Bertrand (1914). *Ibid.* XXVIII. 121.

Bertrand and Berthelot (1913). *Lancet*, p. 523.

Bienstock (1884). *Zeit. f. klin. Med.* VIII. 1.

—— (1899). *Archiv f. Hygiene*, XXXVI. 335.

—— (1901). *Ibid.* XXXIX. 390.

—— (1906). *Ann. de l'Inst. Pasteur*, XX. 497.

Bierotte and Machida (1910). *Münch. med. Woch.* LVII. 636.

Booker (1897). *Johns Hopkins Hosp. Reports*, VI. 159.

Cantu (1911). *Ann. de l'Inst. Pasteur*, XXV. 852.

Dale and Laidlaw (1911). *Journ. of Physiol.* XLIII. 182.

Delépine (1903). *Journ. of Hygiene*, III. 68.

Discussion of Alimentary Toxaemia (1913). Various speakers. *Proc. Roy. Soc. of Med.* Vol. VI. Parts I. and II. No. 5 and No. 7 (supplements).

Ellinger and Gentzen (1903). *Hofmeister's Beitrag*, IV. 171.

Glücksmann (1899). *Centralb. f. Bakt.* I Abt. XXV. 696.

Groot (1918). *Ann. de l'Inst. Pasteur*, XXXII. 299.

Halliburton (1916). *Essentials of Chemical Physiology*, 9th Edition.

Herter (1907). *The common bacterial infections of the digestive tract.* New York.

Herter and Broeck (1911). *Journ. of Biol. Chem.* IX. 491.

Herter and Wakeman (1899). *Journ. of Exp. Med.* IV. 307.

Hopkins and Cole (1903). *Journ. of Physiol.* XXIX. 451.

Horowitz (1916). *Ann. de l'Inst. Pasteur*, XXX. 307.

122   PUTREFACTION   [CH.

Jensen (1903). *"Kalbërruhr,"* Kolle und Wassermann, *Handbuch der Pathogenen Microorg.* III. 779.

Klein (1890). *Report of Medical Officer, Local Gov. Board for 1890*, p. 196.

Ledingham (1913). *Brit. Med. Journ.* I. 821.

Levy (1894). *Archiv f. Exp. Path. u. Pharm.* XXXIV. 342.

Levy and Thomas (1895). *Ibid.* XXXV. 109.

Mandel (1912). *Centralb. f. Bakt.* 1 Abt. Orig. LXVI. 194.

Martin (1901–2). *Med. Officer's Report, Loc. Gov. Board*, 1901–2, p. 395.

—— (1902–3). *Ibid.* 1902–3, p. 496.

—— (1903–4). *Ibid.* 1903–4, p. 461.

McIntosh (1917). *Special Report No.* 12 *Medical Research Committee.*

Mellanby and Twort (1911). *Lancet*, II. 8.

Metchnikoff (1914). *Ann. de l'Inst. Pasteur*, XXVIII. 80.

Ohlmacher (1902). *Journ. of Med. Research*, VII. 411.

Passini (1905). *Zeit. f. Hyg.* XLIX. 135.

Pauly (1917). *Münch. med. Woch.* LXIV. 377.

Pergola (1910). *Centralb. f. Bakt.* 1 Abt. Orig. LIV. 418.

—— (1912). *Ibid.* LXIII. 193.

Pfuhl (1900). *Zeit. f. Hyg.* XXXV. 265.

Plimmer (1912). *The chemical constitution of the proteins*, I.

Rettger (1906). *Journ. of Biol. Chem.* II. 71.

—— (1908). *Ibid.* IV. 45.

—— and Newell (1912–13). *Journ. of Biol. Chem.* XIII. 341.

Rettger, Berman and Sturges (1916). *Journ. of Bact.* I. 15.

Robertson (1918). *Brit. Med. Journ.* I. 583.

Sacquépée and Loygue (1914). *Compt. rend. de la Soc. de Biologie*, LXXVI. 820.

Schellhorn (1910). *Centralb. f. Bakt.* 1 Abt. Orig. LIV. 428.

Schumburg (1902). *Zeit. f. Hyg.* XLI. 183.

Silberschmidt (1898). *Zeit. f. Hyg.* XXX. 328.

Smith, Theobald (1894). *Trans. Ass. of Am. Phys.* IX. 85.

Sperry and Rettger (1915). *Journ. Biol. Chem.* XX. 445.

Tissier (1912). *Ann. de l'Inst. Pasteur*, XXVI. 522.

Tissier and Martelly (1902). *Ann. de l'Inst. Pasteur*, XVI. 865.

Van Loghem and Loghem-Pouw (1912). *Centralb. f. Bakt.* Orig. LXVI. 19.

Van Slyke and Hart (1903). *Amer. Chem. Journ.* XXIX. 150.

Vaughan (1913). V. C. Vaughan, V. C. Vaughan, junr, and J. W. Vaughan, *Protein Split Products*, 1913.

Vaughan and Novy (1903). *Cellular Toxins*, 4th Edition.

Vincent (1909). *Bull. de l'Acad. de Méd.* LXII. 338.

Wells (1914). *Chemical Pathology*, 2nd Edition.

Wesenberg (1898). *Zeit. f. Hyg.* XXVIII. 484.

Zweifel (1911). *Centralb. f. Bakt.* 1 Abt. Orig. LVIII. 115.

ADDENDUM IV.

NOTES ON THE DISTRIBUTION AND PATHOGENICITY OF *B. PROTEUS*.

The earlier accounts give this organism, or rather group of organisms, a very wide distribution in nature under saprophytic conditions. *Proteus vulgaris* is said to be very common in soil, contaminated water, in most decomposing and decaying substances and to be a frequent inhabitant of the animal intestine. The group of organisms conveniently included under the term *B. proteus* has not been very exactly defined and there is some difference of opinion and practice as to the organisms to be included under this designation.

Cantu (1911) carried out an extensive investigation upon the distribution of *B. proteus* in nature, examining rather over 2000 samples from different sources. Unfortunately he does not state clearly the amounts of each substance examined, so the results are not particularly conclusive. The greatest prevalence (20 per cent. or over) was found in the following:

Material	Number of samples examined	Number in which *B. proteus* found	Percentage prevalence
Tainted meat	22	22	100
Dung	25	20	80
Excreta of poultry on a meat diet	30	20	66·6
Garden soil	52	23	44·2
Human excreta: diarrhoea cases	40	16	40
Uncooked sausage	30	10	33·3
Melons	30	7	23·3
Salad	20	4	20

Fairly prevalent also on celery (17·5 per cent.), banana (15 per cent.), cheese (15 per cent.), mouth cavity (12·5 per cent.), flies from dung (12 per cent.).

On the other hand this organism was only found in seven out of 200 samples of milk, once out of 190 samples of air, absent from 100 bread samples, once out of eighty samples of drinking water and absent from ninety samples of ice. The distribution was very variable as out of 392 samples of raisins, prunes, grapes and pears it was not found once, while prevalent on melons and bananas.

Groot (1918) using the same method as Cantu obtained the following results:

Material	Number of samples	Number with *Proteus*	Percentage positive
Adult excreta or intestinal contents	22	8	36
Putrefactive meat	8	8	100
Garden soil	7	4	57
Nursing infants' excreta	26	14	54
Excreta of older children	23	2	8·5

The prevalence on meat foods was also shown by Zweifel (1911), who examined 248 samples of Leipzig "hackfleisch" obtained quite fresh, from which he isolated Proteus bacilli in 165 cases (66 per cent.). All the strains were non-pathogenic to mice by feeding.

Sacquépée and Loygue (1914) examined fifty samples of sausages, ham, pork pies, etc., and found these bacilli present in eighteen cases (36 per cent.).

Bierotte and Machida (1910) investigating the germ content of the organs of quite healthy domestic animals found *Proteus vulgaris* twice in fifty-four organs from eleven animals.

The writer has specially examined a considerable number of samples of garden soil and the excreta of healthy animals for these bacilli and has failed to find them in most cases, and is inclined to think them not so widespread as is supposed. On the other hand, they can almost invariably be found in meat after the onset of putrefactive changes.

In pathological conditions, apart from food poisoning, *B. proteus* has been given a considerable disease-producing rôle by a number of investigators. Jensen considers this organism to be the cause of some forms of calf dysentery. Jaeger came to the conclusion that Weil's disease (infectious jaundice), an acute infectious disease characterised by jaundice, was due to a variety of *B. proteus*, a view supported by other investigators. *B. proteus* has been established as a rare cause of suppuration of various kinds in man, and it must be considered as a feebly pyrogenic bacillus. Pauly (1917) has recently given a number of such instances.

The most important disease for which this organism has been advanced as being etiologically connected is epidemic infantile diarrhoea. Of earlier writers Booker (1897) and also Jeffries and Baginsky concluded that *Proteus vulgaris* and other organisms played a part in the condition, but they did not suggest this organism as the sole cause.

This conception was revived by Metchnikoff and his school. Metchnikoff in 1914 summed up his conclusions as follows: "The chief microbe in the diarrhoea of nurslings is *Proteus*. Its presence is nearly constant in our cases of this disease, also its pathogenic rôle when administered by the mouth, either alone or associated with other microbes, demonstrates its preponderating importance."

While this conclusion is by no means accepted generally, undoubtedly, according to this French school, *B. proteus* does seem to be abundantly present in this condition. For example, Metchnikoff, during 1910 and 1913, investigated bacteriologically 218 cases and isolated Proteus from 204 of them (93·6 per cent.). Bertrand (1914) in fifty-five cases of infantile diarrhoea found *Proteus vulgaris* in every case, while he only isolated this bacillus in two out of twenty-four samples of excreta from infants suffering from diseases other than that of the alimentary canal. Horowitz (1916) investigated an epidemic of acute gastro-enteritis in Petrograd in August, 1913, and studied sixty-three cases, finding *B. proteus* in twenty-four (38 per cent.). The strains isolated showed high virulence to guinea-pigs by intra-peritoneal injection but were without effect when fed.

A number of earlier investigators have shown that *B. proteus* may be possessed of considerable pathogenicity when injected into small rodents. From the different experiments it would appear that this organism is one with very varying virulence, that any toxic symptoms are essentially in proportion to the dose and that pathogenic effects are usually, but not invariably, due to toxins produced outside the body rather than to a true infection. Comparatively few feeding experiments appear to have been made with this organism, and the results are very conflicting. The following may be mentioned in addition to those referred to under the individual outbreaks recorded in Addendum V.

Sidney Martin (1901–04) carried out a series of investigations upon the products of *Proteus vulgaris*. He found a toxic substance in the bodies of this bacillus readily extracted from the dried bodies by distilled water. The physiological action of this substance in fatal or moderate doses was the production of a great lowering of body temperature in the rabbit, sometimes over 7° Fahr., the production of rapid evacuation of the intestinal contents and the causation of great bodily weakness, in some cases followed by collapse and death. This toxic body was found in the filtrate of broth cultures, diminishing in those over two weeks old, and is an excretion of the bacillus. It was not completely destroyed by heat, but the physiological effect was weakened.

Other products of this organism, which are more correctly described as putrefactive products, such as the aromatic alcoholic extract, and the foul smelling bodies which are removed by distillation, have but a slight physiological action.

Unfortunately Martin does not appear to have carried out any feeding experiments, and his investigations throw little light upon the power of *B. proteus* to produce toxins which can cause diarrhoea by feeding.

Metchnikoff (1914) gave a young chimpanzee by the mouth several culture tubes of *B. proteus*, isolated from an infant suffering from diarrhoea, and the animal suffered from gastro-enteritis and died after four days, with abundance of *B. proteus* in the alimentary tract. Nursing rabbits a few days old were fed with *B. proteus* in broth and white of egg and a number of them died, i.e. twenty-two out of thirty-seven. The signs were those of experimental cholera and only one rabbit showed diarrhoea. Experiments with such young animals are not however very impressive.

Herter and Broeck (1911) carried out a few feeding experiments with two strains of *B. proteus vulgaris*. Young guinea-pigs and nursing kittens were unaffected. Of three monkeys (*Macacus rhesus*) fed daily with 50 c.c. of broth cultures, two were unaffected even after a month's feeding, while the third showed diarrhoea with green stools. After 1½ months the animal became very weak and was killed. The walls of the large intestine were thickened, congested, and showed numerous small ulcerations. Cultures from the spleen and blood were sterile. The blood showed a slight agglutination reaction (1 to 50) to *B. proteus*.

Pergola (1910 and 1912) isolated *B. proteus* from sausages which were associated with a small outbreak of illness at Lugo in Italy. The bacillus isolated was very virulent to guinea-pigs, rabbits, mice and rats, both by inoculation and feeding. In cats the effect was variable. Usually the disease set up was acute, but in some cases protracted infection with subsequent death resulted. Some of the prolonged cases were after feeding. The internal organs were usually sterile but the bacillus set up enteritis and could easily be isolated from the intestinal contents. The outbreak is described in Addendum V.

Berthelot (1914 b) studied the pathogenicity of a strain of proteus obtained from a case of infantile diarrhoea. Subcutaneous injection of broth cultures into guinea-pigs and rabbits caused a local abscess, if the cultures were young, but death if old or if given in large amount. Intraperitoneal or intravenous injections all caused death. Intraperitoneal injections of the living bacterial bodies alone caused death in guinea-pigs and rabbits in amounts equivalent to 2–5 mgrm. of dried microbes, the bacilli being abundant in the heart blood. Seven days' old broth cultures after the bacilli were killed were also always toxic intraperitoneally or intravenously. Unfortunately no feeding experiments were carried out.

It may also be mentioned that Jensen claimed to have set up symptoms of calf dysentery in those animals by feeding them with broth cultures of B. proteus.

A point in regard to the toxicity of B. proteus which may be of considerable importance is the power which it seems to possess of increasing the pathogenicity of other organisms. Levy and Thomas (1895), for example, found that the virulence of the cholera spirillum was raised by injecting cultures of proteus precipitated by alcohol. Vincent (1909) found this organism present in severe cases of typhoid fever and that mixed cultures of proteus and typhoid bacilli were very virulent to rabbits.

On the other hand, Theobald Smith (1894) found when B. suipestifer and proteus were grown together that while the virulence of the latter organism was raised that of B. suipestifer was diminished.

Metchnikoff found that greater pathogenicity to quite young rabbits was shown when they were fed with a mixture of cultures of B. proteus and B. welchii, than when either were fed separately. Similar results were obtained with B. proteus and other organisms and Metchnikoff concluded that the pathogenic action of B. proteus in infantile diarrhoea was increased when acting with some other microbes.

Berthelot (1914 a) following up Metchnikoff's work produced diarrhoea in young rats by feeding them with sterilized milk containing B. proteus and B. aminophilus (a bacillus closely allied to B. lactis aerogenes). B. proteus fed alone set up no symptoms. When infection occurred B. proteus was isolated, in a number of cases, from the heart blood of the rats.

These facts suggest the possibility that any toxic properties of putrefactive meat may be due to a symbiotic action between B. proteus and other aerobic or anaerobic organisms.

ADDENDUM V.

FOOD POISONING OUTBREAKS ASCRIBED TO B. PROTEUS.

A number of food poisoning outbreaks have been definitely ascribed to B. proteus. The following is a brief summary of the most important and most frequently quoted outbreaks:

1. *Outbreak described by Levy* (1894). Eighteen persons who frequented a certain restaurant were suddenly attacked with bloody diarrhoea, vomiting, depression and slight fever. Convalescence was very protracted. Several of the cases were very severe, and one patient died. The incubation period is not stated.

The outbreak was ascribed to B. proteus on the following grounds:

(a) The meat used was stored in a refrigerator. This had a strong odour of decomposition when examined and the floor was covered with a slimy brown crust which had an unpleasant stale odour and contained abundance of B. proteus. Both the raw and the cooked meat were kept for several days in the ice-chest.

(b) In the fatal case proteus bacilli were isolated post mortem from the intestinal contents although *not* from the heart blood.

(c) The proteus bacilli isolated were pathogenic to animals, and when *injected* caused haemorrhagic   noea with the presence of proteus in nearly pure culture in the stoc

(d) The symptoms in the patients and in the inoculated animals were said to be similar. The post mortem findings in the fatal case were similar to those shown in animals killed by sepsin.

It will be noted that no proof is advanced that B. proteus was present in or on the actual food eaten (this was, presumably, not examined); that the bacillus was not isolated from the fatal case apart from the intestine, the latter fact being of small significance since this organism is sometimes a natural intestinal inhabitant, and that no animal-feeding experiments were carried out.

The outbreak is apparently ascribed to B. proteus because such bacilli virulent on *injection* into laboratory animals were found in a situation where they could have contaminated the food which caused the outbreak. In view of the wide distribution of proteus this is wholly insufficient evidence.

2. *Mansfield. In August, 1897. Described by Wesenberg* (1898). Sixty-three persons were attacked after eating chopped-up meat derived from an emergency-slaughtered cow, the meat being eaten either raw or in the form of slightly-cooked liver. The cow suffered from a traumatic pericardial inflammation. The meat had been stored in a very damp cellar and piled up piece upon piece. It showed commencing decomposition.

A proteus bacillus was isolated from the meat, but as the latter already showed marked decomposition when it reached the laboratory this is not surprising. This bacillus when *injected* into mice and guinea-pigs was virulent.

Those who had eaten the food after cooking remained unaffected. The symptoms were diarrhoea, headache, body pains, muscular weakness, vertigo and faintness. All recovered.

Here the diagnosis of proteus as the cause is based upon finding it in the meat in a condition which proved virulent on inoculation.

3. *Outbreak in March, 1898 described by Glücksmann* (1899). Two persons (father and son) fell ill a few hours after eating a little half-smoked pork derived from a pig slaughtered on account of disease (nature not ascertained). One of the patients died.

The smoked meat was only examined four days after the fatal meal, and it had then undergone decomposition. When examined, colonies of B. proteus vulgaris were very abundant. Broth cultures of the isolated proteus *injected* into mice and guinea-pigs killed them with symptoms of diarrhoea.

Here, of course, there is no evidence at all of a proteus infection.

4. *Outbreak in Switzerland described by Silberschmidt* (1898). In September, 1898. Forty-five cases due to the consumption of one kind of sausage (so-called "Landjäger"). The symptoms, for the most part, came on about twenty-four hours after eating. The chief symptoms were very profuse diarrhoea, severe cramp-like body pains, fever—often marked—vomiting in most cases and marked prostration. The duration of the disease was considerable, most of the cases being about two weeks under treatment. One death occurred, two and a half days after eating. No bacteriological investigation of the patients was made. Apart from a rancid taste, the sausage meat appeared normal. B. proteus vulgaris and a coli-like bacillus were isolated from the sausage meat.

Some feeding experiments were made, but they were quite inconclusive. Mice and guinea-pigs fed with dry pieces of sausage were unaffected, but when pieces of the sausage were kept for several days in broth and then fed to mice and guinea-pigs, the latter died and B. *proteus* was isolated from the intestinal content, but not from the organs.

Here, obviously, there is no evidence that proteus was the cause of the outbreak.

5. *Hanover. Described by Pfuhl* (1900). During the night of April 12th, 1900, eighty-one soldiers were suddenly attacked with acute gastro-enteritis, four to twelve hours after eating sausage meat. The symptoms rapidly subsided.

The sausage meat was not packed into skins, but into jars. It was prepared on April 11th from heart, lungs and stomach of three different animals. It was cooled in the preparation-room. The sausage meat, in appearance, taste and smell, was perfectly normal. No evidence of putre-factive products could be obtained by injecting animals with alcoholic and ether extracts. No information was available as to the health of the animals.

The bacteriological examination of the sausage meat showed, in addition to other bacteria, B. *proteus* in abundance.

Two rats and two mice were fed with the sausage. The rats each received about ten grammes and were ill, suffering from diarrhoea, but recovered. The mice received about five grammes and were also ill with diarrhoea. One was killed twenty-four hours after feeding and B. *proteus* (*P. mirabile* Hauser) was isolated from the blood and internal organs, cocci and a sarcina being also present. The other mouse died three days after feeding, and proteus was isolated from the internal organs. The proteus isolated from this mouse was slightly virulent.

While there is slightly more evidence in this outbreak pointing to proteus toxins as the cause, there is no etiological connection established as the human cases do not appear to have been bacteriologically investigated.

The feeding experiments do not prove much since it is not uncommon to recover B. *proteus*, B. *coli*, etc., from mice which have died after feeding with foods such as sausage meat. Schellhorn (1910), for example, fed a large number of mice with germ-free meat and 50 per cent. died, usually within three to five days. 115 mice died in this way. As a rule no bacilli were found post mortem but in a few cases B. *coli* were found. B. *proteus* was not isolated by him from any of the mice.

The sausage meat in Pfuhl's cases was prepared from stomach, etc., so the presence of proteus in it is of no special significance, and even if the strain present was toxic to mice when administered in sausage meat, this fact would not necessarily indicate an etiological connection between the sausage meat and the outbreak.

On other grounds, it is unlikely that B. *proteus* was the cause of illness in these cases. The rapid onset and quick subsidence point either to chemi-cal poisons or to toxins only. It is improbable that the poisonous elements in this meat were due to B. *proteus*, since the meat was quite healthy in appearance, odour, etc., and there does not appear to have been sufficient time for any products of the kind to be formed.

It is more likely that the outbreak was due to heat-resistant toxins, the product of some other organism, the organism itself having been killed in the process of preparing the sausages. The feeding experiments do not negative this, since the heat-resisting toxins might kill the mice and allow secondary invasion by intestinal bacilli, such as proteus.

The report does not say when the sausage meat was examined. If not examined immediately the presence of proteus is easily accounted for.

6. *Hanover. Described by Schumburg* (1902). In May, 1901, thirty-four persons became ill after eating sausage. The symptoms came on after a few hours and consisted of nausea, profuse diarrhoea, repeated vomiting, weakness and debility. In most of the cases the symptoms subsided after twelve hours, and only in one or two persons did they continue until next day.

The sausage meat was not put into skins but was used loose. When bacteriologically examined it showed two kinds of bacteria—one a member of the potato bacillus group, the other proteus. A rat and two mice fed with the sausage meat died after twenty-four hours and proteus was isolated from the spleen, liver and heart blood, and was abundantly present in the intestinal contents. The strain isolated from these animals was virulent when fed to mice and rats.

Apparently no examinations at all were made of the patients, and the proof rests solely upon finding a *B. proteus* in the food which was virulent to mice and rats.

7. *Ohio, 1897.* Ohlmacher (1902) described an outbreak in November, 1897, affecting 218 inmates of the Ohio Hospital for Epileptics, all of whom were attacked within a period of three days with severe food poisoning symptoms. No deaths although many were severely ill. Only the patients eating in one block of dining rooms were affected and the only article peculiar to these dining rooms was the oatmeal. This oatmeal was prepared by steaming the batch of twenty gallons in three large pans and then allowing it to cool slowly overnight, it being warmed up again in the morning. On the day before the outbreak, owing to repairs being executed, a large quantity of old plaster in the ceiling of the room used for steaming was knocked off and replaced with new, and the pans, being only covered by loosely fitting bins and sheets of paper, must have been infected with abundance of the dust. The oatmeal would be at about body temperature when so infected. A simple bacteriological examination of the plaster dust showed *B. coli communis* and a bacillus closely resembling *Proteus vulgaris*.

Broth tubes inoculated with plaster scrapings and incubated for twenty-four hours gave cultures rapidly fatal to guinea-pigs when injected intra-peritoneally. Freshly-cooked oatmeal infected with plaster dust and incubated for twelve hours caused no appreciable effect when fed to rabbits and cats. The infected oatmeal was treated by the Stass-Otto method for ptomaines but the yellowish oily liquid so obtained had no effect on three cats.

The author only gives a guarded opinion as to the cause of the outbreak but suggests that either of the above bacilli, or both in combination, may have been the cause of the outbreak.

This outbreak is unusual and interesting on that account, but there is no evidence incriminating *B. proteus* and the general particulars given are against any such view. It was quite possibly due to a Gaertner group organism which would easily be overlooked by the simple bacteriological methods used.

8. *Lugo, 1908.* Pergola (1910) studied a small outbreak of food poisoning (number of cases not given) at Lugo, near Ravenna, in May, 1908, following the use of sausages made from pig's meat. From the

sausages he isolated two bacteria, one of which (*B. mesentericus vulgatus*) was non-pathogenic, the other (*B. proteus*) was pathogenic. In a second paper (1912) he discusses the pathogenic properties of this strain of proteus. He made no faeces or vomit examinations, carried out no agglutination tests with the blood of those attacked, made no investigations as to the source of the sausages or possibility of infection, but states that he found no harmful chemical substances in the sausages.

On this extremely slender evidence this outbreak is added to the list of those caused by *B. proteus*.

9. *Outbreak in 1912 described by Mandel.* An outbreak of forty-six cases of food poisoning in a regiment, ascribed to eating stewed fish. No deaths. None of the fish was available for bacteriological examination, but the stools of twenty-eight cases were examined. From a number of them, seven in almost pure culture, Mandel (1912) isolated bacilli which he describes as *B. proteus vulgaris*. The organisms isolated were not all identical and do not agree in all characters with this organism.

The sera of a number of the patients were tested against the isolated organism and ten of them gave a distinct positive reaction (macroscopic) in a dilution of 1 in 25. A similar positive reaction was given by one of the cases which showed no proteus strains in the excreta and by one of the cooks who was bacteriologically negative, and who was not attacked. The diagnosis of *B. proteus* infection is based upon these bacteriological findings and while more decisive than in most of the above cases cannot be said to supply definite or satisfactory proof.

From this summary of outbreaks it is evident that for none of them was it established that *B. proteus* was etiologically concerned.

CHAPTER VIII

CERTAIN SPECIAL KINDS OF FOOD POISONING

In general, food poisoning outbreaks are more conveniently grouped according to their bacterial origin rather than in relation to the kind of food infected. Certain kinds of food poisoning are, however, on account of their special nature, more conveniently studied from the food standpoint. These will be briefly considered in the present section.

Mussel poisoning.

Epidemics of typhoid fever have been frequently traced to the consumption of mussels as well as to other shellfish. In addition to these epidemics outbreaks of acute poisoning attributed to the consumption of mussels have been recorded on numerous occasions.

In the recorded outbreaks the onset has usually been rapid and within a few hours of consuming the mussels, but occasionally it has been delayed for even as long as eighteen to twenty-four hours. While the ordinary food poisoning symptoms are met with to some· extent, i.e. vomiting, diarrhoea and epigastric pain, they may be absent, and only very rarely are dominant symptoms. The main symptoms are referable to the nervous system. In the Leith outbreak, for example, Combe, who described it, gives the chief symptoms as—prickly feeling in the hands and feet, feeling of constriction of the mouth and throat, difficulty in swallowing and speaking freely, numbness about the mouth, gradually extending to the arms, and muscular weakness of the limbs.

In the Dublin cases, described by Sir Charles Cameron, the chief symptoms were vomiting, dyspnoea, swelling of the face, want of co-ordination of movement, spasms, especially of the arms. The onset started with prickly pains in the hands.

Almost identical symptoms were described by Schmidt-mann in cases observed by him in some workmen and members of their families who had eaten mussels obtained from a newly constructed dock. In these cases there was no abdominal pain or diarrhoea, but nausea and vomiting occurred. One person died in $1\frac{3}{4}$ hours, another after $3\frac{1}{2}$ hours and a third five hours after eating the mussels.

In a case described by Hill (1895) the symptoms came on almost immediately after eating the mussels and death after about an hour.

The symptoms are often very severe and not infrequently fatal, as shown in the following particulars of a few outbreaks in the British Isles:

Place	Date	Number of Cases	Number of Deaths
Leith	1827	30	2
Liverpool	1872	2	1
Ramsgate	1880	2	0
Liverpool	1888	3	1
Dublin	1890	7	5
Barry	1909	19	1
		63	10

Case mortality, 16 per cent.

Many explanations have been advanced to account for the causation of mussel poisoning. These are carefully reviewed by Bulstrode in his report (1894–5) to the Local Government Board on "Oyster Culture in relation to Disease." The earlier views ascribing the pathogenic properties to copper poisoning, starfish spawn, mussels eaten during the spawning season, mussels eaten in a stale or dead condition, may be dismissed as untrue or inadequate as explanations generally applicable although metallic poisoning cannot be excluded as a possible cause of illness in individual cases or even in small outbreaks.

The Wilhelmshaven cases directed attention into another field. From a number of the poisonous mussels Brieger obtained a poisonous base, which he regarded as a ptomaine, and called *mytilotoxine*. The symptoms produced in animals by the injection of this substance are, according to Brieger, similar to those produced in mussel poisoning.

Salkowski (1885) found that the toxic substance was not destroyed by current steam.

When mussels have caused illness it has invariably been found that they were taken from positions liable to sewage pollution, such as from dock walls or vessels in harbours. Although in opposition to this there is the undoubted fact that very large numbers of this shellfish, taken from sources equally exposed to sewage pollution, are eaten without harm, it is highly probable that their toxic properties are derived from their polluted surroundings. Schmidtmann, for example, found that healthy non-poisonous mussels placed in polluted water from which poisonous mussels were obtained themselves became poisonous, while the harmful mussels kept in clear running sea-water became non-toxic.

No modern investigations appear to have been made upon the bacteria causing poisonous properties in mussels, but McWeeney (1890), published some preliminary investigations and quotes Lustig as having, in 1888, isolated from the livers of specimens of mussels a bacillus rapidly pathogenic to rabbits and guinea-pigs.

The rapidity of onset and (when fatal) rapidly fatal result make it evident that the symptoms are due to a chemical poison, while the peculiar symptoms differentiate this type from the ordinary food poisoning outbreaks.

The most probable view is that mussels become poisonous from the production in them of chemical poisons elaborated by the vital activity of bacteria derived from their sewage contaminated surroundings, but we are ignorant of the special bacteria concerned, the conditions which cause the production of these poisons, and whether the toxic properties are due to mytilotoxine or to some other bacterial poisons.

Very few outbreaks appear to have been reported in recent years, but it is desirable that the whole subject should be re-investigated by modern methods.

Poisoning from other kinds of shellfish.

Oysters eaten out of the season are said to cause gastro-enteritis, urticaria, and other symptoms, but acute and intense poisoning of the type recorded under mussel poisoning appears to be rare. Two instances may be mentioned in both of which one or more of the oysters appeared not to have been perfectly healthy judged by the senses.

In the case recorded by Casey (1894) a man ate eight oysters for supper, remarking at the time that one of them was bad. Others of the same lot were eaten by other persons with impunity and appeared to be quite fresh. The symptoms commenced about twelve or fourteen hours after the meal with pains in the back, violent abdominal pain, frequent vomiting and intense thirst; there was no diarrhoea. Later the patient collapsed and died forty-one hours after eating the oysters.

Brosch (quoted by Novy) reported the case of an officer who died in twelve hours after eating some oysters which at the time were noticed to possess a bad taste. The symptoms began in a few hours and were more like those of botulism than mussel poisoning.

Lobsters have been reported on several occasions as causing outbreaks of severe illness. Novy quotes a case in which a number of young people ate a mayonnaise made from canned lobsters. The symptoms were nausea, vomiting, much pain, severe headache, small, rapid pulse, and a slightly subnormal temperature. Neither urticaria, eye symptoms, nor paralysis occurred.

Although not due to shellfish the case of poisoning from sardines reported by Stevenson (1892) was probably similar in nature. In this case a young officer ate six sardines on toast, from a newly opened tin, for breakfast. He said the fish tasted nasty. At lunch he was unwell and vomited soon afterwards, while more serious symptoms developed later in the day. He died the following day. The sardines were only examined five days after death but were then intensely toxic to rats and mice by feeding.

Galeotti and Zardo (1902) report a considerable outbreak at Isola (Austria) in November, 1900, from the consumption of sea-snails (*Murex bradatus*). All the forty-three persons attacked had eaten sea-snails which three to five days previously had been removed about five miles from the shore.

The symptoms appeared within a short time after consumption of the molusks and were of the usual food poisoning rather than the mussel poisoning type. In certain cases less direct symptoms, such as haematuria, cramps, disturbance of speech, and muscular feebleness were exhibited. Five died but, although post mortems were made, bacteriological investigations were not carried out in these cases nor from the snails actually consumed. From the livers of sea-snails from the same region they subsequently isolated in pure culture a very virulent bacillus, which from the very incomplete description appears to be a variety of *B. coli* or possibly a Gaertner group organism. It was highly pathogenic to guinea-pigs and rabbits by injection and killed rabbits in five to eight days when introduced into the stomach and also when fed to a dog. A year later they isolated what they describe as the same bacillus from snails from the same beds, but these possessed little or no pathogenicity. They take the view that some special unknown conditions had made this strain highly virulent and caused the outbreak. Obviously information upon many points not elucidated in the report is needed before this conclusion can be accepted.

Cheese poisoning.

Outbreaks of sudden illness from the consumption of cheese are not very uncommon, cases being more frequently recorded in the United States, but this is perhaps due to the special attention directed to the subject by Vaughan.

The chief symptoms consist of diarrhoea, vomiting and abdominal pain. There is usually some degree of fever; rigors may be met with and symptoms of collapse are often present. The symptoms appear to vary greatly in severity, sometimes being very severe; no deaths were however recorded in either the Michigan (1883–4) or London (1901) outbreaks.

The Michigan outbreak consisted of about 300 cases caused by the consumption of twelve different cheeses. It is not clear if they were obtained from the same source. The incubation period was mostly 2–4 hours, but in a few cases the symptoms were delayed up to 8–12 hours.

In London (Newman, 1901) a considerable outbreak occurred in 1901, the cases being rather scattered: seventeen were traced in Finsbury, twenty-one in Bermondsey, and others in different parts. The symptoms came on from two to eight hours after eating the cheese which was "Dutch cheese," and all made by one firm in Holland. In this outbreak, as in others, the cheese was normal as regards taste, odour and appearance.

The first scientific contribution to the causation of cheese poisoning was made by Vaughan in connection with the above-mentioned Michigan outbreak. From the aqueous extract of the cheese specimens Vaughan separated a crystalline poisonous body which he called *tyro-toxicon*. Tyrotoxicon is not an alkaloid, but in its chemical reactions, and to some extent in its physiological action, resembles diazobenzene.

This substance has since been isolated on a number of occasions from cheese which has caused outbreaks of poisoning. In the London outbreak, mentioned above, the analyst who examined the cheese reported that he obtained a small amount of a body possessing the chief characteristics of tyro-toxicon, but this was only obtained from two out of four samples and then in small quantity only. Two other chemists examined samples but failed to isolate this poison.

In this outbreak more than seventy cheeses were purchased by the wholesale firm and positive evidence of poisoning was forthcoming for only a few of them. A bacteriological examination by Klein yielded no definite results. Although small quantities of tyro-toxicon were found and the outbreak was ascribed to this cause, the evidence recorded does not satisfactorily prove this contention since it rests upon the fact that one analyst out of three, in two out of four samples, found quite small quantities of a body possessing the characteristics of tyro-toxicon. The bacteriological investigations showed the presence of *B. coli communis, Bacterium lactis* and other bacteria, but no bacteriological relationship to the outbreak was disclosed.

Wallace (1887) mentions two outbreaks in America of poisoning associated with the consumption of cheese. In one at Jeanesville in January, 1886, over fifty persons were suddenly taken ill while a similar but less extensive outbreak took place at Riverton some months later. No deaths. Tyro-toxicon was found to be present in both lots of cheese. In the Jeanesville case the cheese causing the illness was one of a lot of thirty all received at the same time from the factory; twenty-seven had been sold and no illness resulted.

Tyro-toxicon has also been isolated from poisonous cheese by Wolff and other investigators.

A rather peculiar outbreak ascribed to cheese poisoning occurred at Aldershot in 1899 (B.M.J. 1899). Between August 26th and September 10th twenty-seven cases occurred with three deaths, the chief symptoms being fever (100°–103° C), vomiting and feeble pulse with, in severe cases, cramps in the calves. When these symptoms persisted for three or four days jaundice occurred in a good many of the cases. The rations included a daily allowance of cheese. Some of the patients however stated that they ate no cheese, while tinned beef and German sausages were also included in the ration. The cheese which was obtained from abroad was not abnormal in appearance or smell while, according to the contractor, it was supplied to other customers without complaint being made or illness resulting. The chief feature of interest in the outbreak is that twenty sheep happened to feed on the camp refuse, including potato peelings, onions, pieces of cheese, etc., and that some eight of them sickened and two died in two to three days. After burial three bodies were exhumed. From pieces of cheese obtained from the stomachs of these animals Luff found tyro-toxicon in fairly large quantity and one milligramme of this body injected into a rat killed it in three hours. Bacteriological examination of the cheese from the sheep by Klein and Wright showed nothing worthy of note.

Later investigations have shown that tyro-toxicon is not present in all poisonous cheeses, and that in such cases at least the harmful properties must be ascribed to other causes.

Vaughan and Novy (1903) state that tyro-toxicon has also been found in milk in numerous instances and mention outbreaks described by Firth in 1887 in India, by Schearer in 1886 and by Vaughan in 1887, in all of which tyro-toxicon was isolated. Wallace also describes an outbreak in which forty-three persons were taken ill and in which tyro-toxicon was isolated from the milk, and mentions a similar outbreak at Memphis. It is significant to note that there are few if any recent references to the finding of tyro-toxicon in cheese and all these reports date from the period when the chemical and ptomaine theory of food poisoning was predominant.

Indeed in some of the more recent outbreaks tyro-toxicon has been looked for but not found. Taltaval and Gies (1907), for example, made a very careful examination of a piece of cheese which had caused decidedly toxic symptoms similar to those described by Vaughan and Novy from poisonous cheese. They failed to find any tyro-toxicon or any alkaloidal substance. Coagulable proteins were absent but tryptophane, leucin, and tyrosine were found and they considered that the poisonous matter was probably due to a toxic proteose.

It may be mentioned as of some interest that Nelson (1916) has demonstrated the presence of indol, skatol, and phenol, in Limburger and Camembert cheese. These protein degradation products were absent from Cheddar, Swiss and other cheeses.

Bacteriological investigations have also been carried out. Vaughan and Perkins (1896) described an outbreak of twelve cases from eating cheese in 1895. From a piece of the cheese they isolated two bacilli, one of which elaborated an active toxin. This bacillus was a strain of *B. coli communis* or *B. lactis aerogenes*, chiefly differing from the former in its more rapid milk clotting power and its failure to produce indol. Both filtered and heated cultures rapidly killed laboratory animals. The toxins were partially heat resistant, not being entirely destroyed by fourteen minutes heating to 100° C.

Owing to a mistake in labelling, the toxicity of a sterilized culture was demonstrated upon a human subject who was made very seriously ill by the injection of ten drops of a concentrated (50 per cent.) germ free milk culture, the symptoms commencing within half an hour.

In subsequent investigations by Vaughan, organisms of the colon group were isolated which produced powerful toxins which were also heat resisting. Thus Vaughan and McClymonds examined sixty-five samples of cheese from as many different manufacturers. Of these forty-nine were American green cheeses. Eight of the forty-nine samples were sent to the laboratory because persons eating them had suffered from nausea, vomiting and purging. The other samples were not known to be poisonous. Every one of the forty-nine samples of American green cheese furnished cultures which killed white rats, guinea-pigs and rabbits, the toxic organisms in all the samples being members of the colon group. The authors record that the cultures could be boiled without destroying their toxicity.

Holst (1896) records five different outbreaks of cheese poisoning observed by him within a period of five months. He isolated *B. coli communis* from each of the five lots of cheese (a Norwegian cheese called "Knet Käse"). He carried out some interesting feeding experiments with quite young calves. When calves were fed with *B. coli* from ordinary sources and from non-poisonous cheese, no diarrhoea or other symptoms were caused, but when calves were fed with the *B. coli* from the cheese—four strains from four separate outbreaks being used in individual experiments— the calves suffered from diarrhoea and in some cases died. In the latter case the bacilli were recovered post mortem from the spleen, blood, etc. The bacilli from the poisonous cheese were also highly virulent to rabbits.

Symanowski (1913) describes an outbreak affecting twenty-seven persons in five households, who were suddenly attacked with vomiting, diarrhoea and colic, and which was due to eating infected cheese bought in the town market. A Gaertner strain (*B. paratyphosus B*) was isolated from the cheese and from the excreta of some of the cases. In addition a number of samples of blood from persons attacked agglutinated this bacillus.

It would appear to be probable that cheese poisoning, like other forms of food poisoning, is usually due to bacteria which produce powerful toxins. The bacterial investigations just recorded suggest that specially virulent strains of *B. coli* are concerned, but further investigation is desirable, and probably in a good many cases Gaertner group bacilli will be found to be the cause, if modern methods of identification are employed.

Ice-cream poisoning.

Although outbreaks of poisoning from eating ice-cream are not infrequent yet, making allowances for the numerous unrecorded cases, they are less numerous than might be anticipated, in view of the unsatisfactory conditions under which much of this food is prepared and the fact that it is a substance which is an admirable nutritive medium for bacteria. It is true that it is subjected in preparation to some degree of heating, but this varies considerably, while the process of cooling afterwards is very slow and prolonged, and being often carried out amidst insanitary surroundings offers abundant facilities for subsequent contamination. Buchan (1910) in Birmingham found that the average duration of cooling after heating was about twenty-one hours. When vended, ice-cream frequently contains from 1 million to 300 million bacteria per cubic centimetre.

Ice-cream has been the vehicle of spread in a number of typhoid fever outbreaks. The one at Eccles (Copeman, 1911) is a good example.

In the series of British outbreaks in Table I six were spread by ice-cream. As an illustration that at Nuneaton in June, 1909, may be quoted. In this outbreak sixty-seven persons were attacked at ages varying from one to fifty years. The ice-cream used was composed of milk, eggs, sugar and gelatine. It was made one evening and allowed to cool (but not frozen) until the next morning when it was ready for sale about 9.30 a.m. It was all eaten that day. The chief symptoms were severe diarrhoea, vomiting and collapse and the incubation period for most cases was from three to nine hours (twenty-four hours in one case). There were no deaths. *B. enteritidis* was isolated from the faeces of one sufferer while the blood serum of another agglutinated this bacillus. No ice-cream was available for examination. In all the six outbreaks only one death was reported.

The earlier observers reported poisonous chemical substances in ice-cream. Thus Vaughan and Novy found tyrotoxicon in several samples of poisonous ice-cream and custard, Schearer reported the same substance in both vanilla and lemon ice-cream which had caused poisoning symptoms, while in 1896 Vaughan and Perkins reported the detection of another toxin in both ice-cream and cheese which had caused illness (about fifty cases from the ice-cream).

Although frequently grouped as a special class of food poisoning, ice-cream outbreaks do not differ in any essential particular from those due to the consumption of other foods and there is no scientific justification for retaining them as a special group. No further details therefore need be given.

Potato poisoning.

A considerable number of outbreaks of food poisoning has been reported from the consumption of potatoes. Earlier investigators, obsessed with the ptomaine theory of meat poisoning and failing to find any source of ptomaines in potatoes, fell back upon chemical instead of animal alkaloids as the source of the mischief and ascribed the symptoms to solanine poisoning. The symptoms produced by solanine are said to be very similar to those of saponine, one of the ptomaines isolated from meat.

Dixon Mann (1908) gives the chief symptoms of poisoning by berries containing solanine as vomiting and diarrhoea, with more or less collapse, pain in the stomach, cramps in the legs followed by clonic spasms, dilatation of the pupils, pallor, coldness of the surface, hallucinations and coma. Morris (1859), for example, gives particulars of a case with somewhat similar symptoms in a girl of fourteen who ate a number of potato berries with a fatal result three days later. The symptoms started a few hours after their consumption.

With a chemical causation in fashion as the explanation of potato poisoning considerable attention was directed to the solanine content of potatoes causing disease symptoms, and it soon became evident that the amounts of this alkaloid present were quite insufficient to produce the symptoms, and indeed in some cases were less than in ordinary healthy potatoes.

Meyer (1895), for example, found the solanine content of potatoes to vary from 0·04 to 0·116 grm. per kilo according to the time of the year, while some young potatoes contained as much as 0·236 grm. per kilo. Potato sprouts and young green potatoes are rich in solanine and Meyer found as much as 0·580 grm. per kilo in little dwarf potatoes budded from old seed potatoes. Esser (1910) states that in midsummer the haulm contains 0·0925 per cent. of solanine, but late in summer only 0·0374 per cent. He also found variations according to the nature of the soil.

On the other hand Dieudonné (1904) found only 0·012 grm. per kilo of solanine in potatoes suspected of having caused an outbreak of food poisoning.

The dose of solanine necessary to produce symptoms of poisoning is not less than 0·2 to 0·4 grm. per kilo. Haselberg (1909) gave this alkaloid in considerably higher doses than this without any symptoms being caused. This writer records that the highest percentage of solanine he has found recorded in any potato poisoning outbreaks was in Weimar in 1897 when 0·426 per cent. of solanine was found. He remarks that perhaps this might be sufficient to produce poisonous symptoms if it can be assumed that at least 1 kilo of potato was taken and that all was absorbed.

Schmiedeberg (1895) suggested that the amount of solanine was increased by bacterial action, while Weil (1900) found that two out of thirteen bacteria investigated by him increased the percentage of solanine. This observation seems unlikely and was not confirmed by Wintgen (1906).

It may be mentioned that Long (1917) records a number of cases of poisoning of animals (horses, pigs, cows) from eating stocks of potatoes, but the symptoms he records are quite different from those which occur in human outbreaks. In these cases, since the quantities of potatoes eaten are so much larger, it is possible that the causation of the symptoms may be due to this alkaloid, particularly since in a number of cases sprouted potatoes, which contain a higher proportion of the alkaloid than ordinary potatoes, were consumed.

On the whole it seems very doubtful if potato poisoning in man is ever caused by solanine poisoning, but the above particulars are interesting as showing how far a preconceived theory may be pushed to elucidate facts.

One of the earliest outbreaks in Great Britain reported from eating potatoes is that described by Banks (1846). The potatoes were eaten for several meals by a family of seven persons, four of whom were attacked with severe symptoms, the most prominent being severe abdominal pain greatly increased by pressure, great tenderness of the rectum and anus, very pronounced constipation, nearly complete suppression of urine and symptoms of collapse. No narcotic symptoms were exhibited, neither were they those of ordinary cases of food poisoning. All recovered, but after a prolonged convalescence. A number of the potatoes exhibited black spots and fibres in their structure, and the father attributes the immunity of the other three cases to their having peeled the potatoes and removed the bad parts, a precaution which those attacked neglected to take. Banks considered that the outbreak was due to the consumption of potatoes in large quantities far advanced in decay. The outbreak was a peculiar one and was probably due to rather gross contamination, probably from fungi, and of a kind not now likely to be met with.

The majority of the more recent investigations suggest that the poisonous symptoms are due to bacterial activity.

Dieudonné (1904) described an extensive outbreak at Hammelburg in August, 1903, when 150 to 180 soldiers became ill two hours after dinner, the symptoms being of sudden onset and consisting of severe vomiting, intense diarrhoea, headache, collapse, etc. The symptoms began to subside after about seven hours in most cases and all ultimately recovered. The outbreak was ascribed to potato salad and from this Dieudonné isolated B. proteus. This bacillus was not virulent in pure culture but when mice were fed with previously sterile potato inoculated with this bacillus and grown for twenty-four hours at 37° C. they died in twenty-four to forty-eight hours. Mice fed with the salad died in twenty-four hours with severe gastro-intestinal symptoms.

In considering these outbreaks three facts are noticeable. In the first place the symptoms are those met with in ordinary outbreaks of food poisoning from infected meat, milk, etc., and are not distinctive as in mussel poisoning.

In the second place it is noteworthy that a large proportion have occurred amongst troops. Cortial (1889), for example, records an outbreak affecting 101 soldiers. Schmiedeberg (1895) gives particulars of four outbreaks all amongst troops in garrisons, one affecting 357 soldiers, one 90, a third 125, and a fourth 43 men. All the 716 men so attacked recovered.

Pfuhl in 1899 described an outbreak affecting fifty-six soldiers ascribed to the eating of salted potatoes. In this instance the peeled potatoes contained 0·038 per cent. solanine when raw and 0·024 per cent. after being boiled. On an average Pfuhl considered that every man who fell ill had 0·3 grm. of the alkaloid, a quantity which he considered sufficient to produce toxic results.

The third distinctive point is the frequency with which the potatoes after peeling were kept in this condition until next day, or at least for a considerable interval, before cooking. The skins of unpeeled potatoes protect them from bacterial infection, but, as is well known, peeled potatoes are valuable nutrient media for bacteria. It is to this factor, and the accompanying specific bacterial infection, and not to any excess of solanine, that the frequency of potatoes as a cause of food poisoning is to be ascribed. For example, in the outbreak recorded by Pfuhl the potatoes concerned were peeled, placed in a vessel filled with water, and remained standing in the water until next day (in May). They were then washed and cooked for twenty-five minutes.

In Dieudonné's outbreak the potatoes were boiled the night preceding the meal, then peeled and kept in this unprotected condition until the next day (in August) in baskets adjoining the camp kitchen. Dieudonné indeed quotes a very interesting instance in which the members of one company of a particular battalion became ill after eating potato salad which had been standing for twenty-four hours, while several other companies had two hours earlier eaten part of the same batch of potatoes without any untoward results.

The only outbreak in England which the writer has come across is one at Norbiton (No. 70 in the series) in August, 1910, and which after a careful study of the available facts he considers was probably due to potato poisoning. As no bacteriological examination of the potatoes was made it is impossible to be certain on this point. Potatoes were the only article eaten in common by all the sufferers. The persons attacked numbered 80 to 100, all having consumed their food at a fried fish shop, the meal being for the most part potatoes and fish fried in oil. The potatoes as purchased were good since half of them, cooked the evening before, were eaten without harm. The remaining half were washed and scrubbed, and left ready for frying on the following day. In this unprotected state they were probably infected in some unascertained way. This inoculated nutrient medium was kept for at least sixteen to twenty hours in a hot shop (in August) and was then fried with the fish. Probably the cooking in the oil killed the bacteria and left their toxins. No one appears to have asked or recorded whether the potatoes appeared good in the morning when they were used and no bacteriological examinations were made.

Harris and Cockburn (1918) have recently re-investigated this subject in connection with an outbreak of food poisoning in Glasgow in November, 1917. From their tabular statement it would appear that sixty-one persons were attacked between November 23rd and 27th, of whom one died (aged five years) after an illness of thirty-one hours. In ten cases the illness lasted for two to three days, but for the remainder only for a few hours. The essential symptoms were headache, vomiting, diarrhoea and debility. The fatal case showed no indications of irritant poisoning and the immediate cause of death was due to strangulation of the bowel, a condition which it was suggested was due to extreme retching and vomiting.

All the persons affected had partaken of potatoes from one source. The potatoes were normal in appearance and were part of a consignment of thirteen truck loads. The buds on quite a number of the potatoes showed evidence of sprouting, being about ¼ inch in length, and their solanine content was estimated.

The samples of potatoes from the household in which the fatal case occurred showed 0·041 per cent. of solanine, while a sample from the store and supposed to be from the same consignment gave 0·0079 per cent. No information is given as to the solanine content of the potatoes consumed by other persons who were attacked.

Bacteriological examination of the potatoes and also of organs from the fatal case gave negative results. The potatoes bacteriologically examined were from the household of the fatal case, but apparently were not part of the potatoes actually consumed.

The contention of the authors that the outbreak was undoubtedly due to solanine poisoning is not completely justified, or at least not proved. The potatoes were part of a large consignment most of which was eaten without any symptoms of poisoning, and which from the single analysis quoted appeared to have the ordinary low solanine content of potatoes. No evidence is submitted that the cases of poisoning coincided with instances in which the potatoes were eaten after sprouting and so presumably in a condition with a high solanine content. The analysis of potatoes from the household with the fatal case gives, it is true, a very high solanine content, but the report is by no means clear that the potatoes actually eaten were in this sprouting condition and says nothing as to whether other persons in this household consumed them without ill effects. The symptoms were not those of poisoning by solanine as described above.

REFERENCES.

Shellfish poisoning.

Brieger (1889). *Virchow's Archiv*, cxv. 483.

Bulstrode. *Supplement to the Medical Officer's Report L.G.B.* 1894–5.

—— (1911). *Report of Medical Officer of L.G.B. for* 1909–10.

Cameron (1890). *Brit. Med. Journ.* II. 150.
Casey (1894). *Ibid.* I. 463.
Combe (1828). *Medical and Surgical Review*, XXIV.
Galeotti and Zardo (1902). *Centralb. f. Bakt.* Orig. XXXI. 593.
Hill (1895). *Brit. Med. Journ.* I. 301.
König. *Nahr. Genussen*, II. 103.
McWeeney (1890). *Brit. Med. Journ.* II. 628.
Neale (1909). *Ibid.* II. 176.
Novy (1915). *Osler and McCrae's System of Medicine*, II. 450.
Permewan (1888). *Lancet*, II. 568.
Salkowski (1885). *Virchow's Archiv*, CII. 578.
Stevenson (1892). *Brit. Med. Journ.* II. 1326.

Examples of mussel poisoning are also given in
Brit. Med. Journ. (1857). Aug. 1st, 657.
Ibid. (1872), II. 592.
Ibid. (1891), II. 749.

Cheese poisoning.

Holst (1896). *Centralb. f. Bakt.* I. Abt. XX. 160.
Nelson (1916). *Journ. Biol. Chem.* XXIV. 533.
Newman (1901). *Report of M.O.H. on Public Health of Finsbury*, 110.
Symanowski (1913). *Zeit. f. Medizinalbeamte*, September 20th, No. 18.
Taltaval and Gies (1907). *New York Med. Journ.* LXXXVI. 726.
Vaughan and Novy (1903). *Cellular Toxins.*
Vaughan and Perkins (1896). *Archiv f. Hyg.* XXVII. 308.
Wallace (1887). *Medical News*, LI. 69.
—— (1899). *Brit. Med. Journ.* II. 1300.

Ice-cream poisoning.

Buchan (1910). *Journ. of Hygiene*, X. 93.
Copeman (1911). *Report to L.G.B.* New Series, No. 51.
Savage (1913). *Ibid.* No. 77. (Food Reports, No. 18.)
Vaughan and Novy (1903). *Cellular Toxins.*
—— and Perkins (1896). *Archiv f. Hyg.* XXVII. 308.

Potato poisoning.

Banks (1846). *Dublin Journ. of Medical Science*, I. (New Series), XXIX. (Old Series), 267.
Cortial (1889). *Arch. de Méd. et de Pharm. Militaire*, XIV. 3.
Dieudonné (1904). *Deut. Militärarztl. Zeit.* XXXIII. 181.
Esser (1910). *Die Giftpflanzen Deutschlands.*
Harris and Cockburn (1918). *The Analyst*, XLIII. 133.
Haselberg (1909). *Medizinische Klinik*, V. 1196.

Long (1917). *Plants poisonous to live stock.*
Mann (Dixon) (1908). *Forensic Medicine and Toxicology.*
Meyer (1895). *Arch. f. exp. Path. u. Pharm.* XXXVI. 375.
Morris (1859). *Brit. Med. Journ.* September 3rd, 719.
Pfuhl (1899). *Deut. med. Woch.* XXV. 753.
Schmiedeberg (1895). *Arch. f. exp. Path. u. Pharm.* XXXVI. 373.
Weil (1900). *Arch. f. Hyg.* XXXVIII. 330.
Wintgen (1906). *Zeit. f. Untersuch. der Nahrungs- und Genussmittel,*
    XII. 113.

CHAPTER IX

BOTULISM

THIS interesting, but fortunately rare, type of food poisoning has been recognized for nearly a century, but knowledge as to its true pathology only dates from 1895. Kerner in 1820 reported upon a number of epidemics in various parts of Würtemberg and in 1822 reported a further ninety-eight cases with thirty-four deaths. Since these dates many other outbreaks have been reported, the greater number of the earlier ones occurring in Würtemberg or its neighbourhood. The majority of these earlier outbreaks were due to eating sausage, and the condition is often spoken of as "sausage poisoning." This name, however, is a very unsuitable one as the condition may be associated with many other kinds of foods. In particular it may be mentioned that a number of outbreaks have occurred in Russia, following the consumption of smoked fish, in which the symptoms bear a close resemblance to botulism and probably were examples of that condition.

Outbreaks of botulism are rather rarely met with at the present time, but in view of the fact that cases of illness have recently occurred in this country which simulated this disease, some detailed consideration is necessary. The writer has been unable to trace the existence of a single definite outbreak in Great Britain. The case recorded by Stephenson (1892) of fatal poisoning of a young man from sardines was evidently due to a bacillus producing very powerful toxins and in some ways resembles this condition, but the recorded symptoms are not those of botulism.

In America Dickson has reported a number of outbreaks and collected instances of others, and in a recent monograph on the subject[1] (Dickson, 1918) he arrives at the conclusion

---

[1] The present chapter was written before this monograph appeared, but it was possible to incorporate a number of interesting points subsequently. Readers desirous of a more complete account of this condition are referred to this valuable monograph.

that botulism is endemic in the United States, and is comparatively common in the Pacific Coast States.

In only a small proportion of the outbreaks recorded as botulism has the specific bacillus described below been isolated, the diagnosis being made upon the clinical data, so that it is desirable to describe the symptoms in some detail. The following account of the symptoms is largely taken from Van Ermengem's monograph upon the subject (Van Ermengem, 1912).

The symptoms exhibited are very characteristic and strikingly different from those met with in ordinary cases of food poisoning. Indeed Van Ermengem states: "The symptoms of botulismus are so uniform and true to nature that for the recognition of the disease clinical appearances alone are sufficient."

The symptoms shown are almost entirely referable to lesions of the central nervous system. Prominent conditions are those referable to disturbance of the digestive tract— such as thirst, feeling of constriction of the throat, dysphagia, skin-like coating of mouth and pharynx, complete loss of appetite, obstinate constipation, and ocular symptoms— such as internal or external and more or less complete ophthalmoplegia, paralysis of accommodation, mydriasis, nystagmus, internal strabismus. Other symptoms which may be met with are diuresis or complete anuria, complete loss of voice, prolapse or paresis of the tongue.

The fatal cases show gradually advancing respiratory and cardiac failure due to progressive bulbar paralysis.

Vomiting and diarrhoea are frequently absent, but may occur and if present are usually slight or transitory. Fever is never observed and indeed the temperature is usually subnormal, muscular cramps do not occur, consciousness is not impaired.

The ocular symptoms usually develop in a progressive order. Amaurosis first occurs, then more or less complete accommodation paralysis frequently followed by ptosis, mydriasis, diplopia, etc. In cases which recover these ocular symptoms may last for many weeks.

The case mortality may be as high as 30 to 50 per cent.,

or even higher, and when death occurs it is usually in the first or second week.

The clinical picture has to be distinguished from polio-encephalitis, bulbar paralysis and the different ophthal-moplegias.

The symptoms usually appear twelve to twenty-four hours after eating the infected food, but now and then are delayed as much as thirty-six to forty-eight hours. Only rarely do they appear earlier than twelve hours.

The recorded pathological lesions in fatal cases are very slight and are chiefly in the direction of hyperaemia of most of the internal organs, and here and there small haemorrhages in the kidneys and spinal cord. Van Ermengem, however, points out that the lesions in man have not been extensively studied, nor by modern methods, and that there can be no doubt that severe and extensive histological changes take place similar to those which occur in animals inoculated with the toxin of *Bacillus botulinus* and which especially manifest themselves in the cerebro-spinal centres.

Dickson (1918) draws attention to the formation of characteristic thrombi and states that they are so uniformly present and are so characteristic in appearance as to be considered pathognomonic of botulism.

The bacterial origin of this variety of food poisoning was first made clear by Van Ermengem, who in 1895 isolated *B. botulinus* from a ham, the consumption of which had caused about thirty cases of botulism at Ellezelles (Belgium) in December of that year. The bacilli, in the form of spores, were present in considerable numbers in the intermuscular connective tissue of one of the three fatal cases and in small numbers in the spleen and contents of the large intestine.

B. botulinus is a large bacillus (4–6 μ long by 0·9 to 1·2 μ wide) which sometimes forms short threads. It is slightly motile with four to eight flagella. Under suitable con-ditions, such as in an alkaline gelatine medium incubated at 20°–25° C., it produces spores which are usually terminal but occasionally central. Spores are not formed at 37° C. The optimum temperature of growth is 20°–30° C. It is gram positive but does not hold the stain strongly.

Growth is scanty in artificial media unless glucose is present or meat is used. It is an obligate anaerobe. Cultures have a rancid butyric acid odour. It liquefies gelatine, ferments glucose (with gas formation), but not saccharose or lactose, the growth in milk is scanty without coagulation or visible change. McIntosh (1917) found that under good anaerobic conditions fair-sized colonies can be obtained in twenty-four hours on serum agar, while coagulated serum is not liquefied. This worker reports slight gas production with lactose and also with maltose, glycerine and starch. The spores are not highly resistant and are destroyed by fifteen minutes at 85° C. or thirty minutes at 80° C. (Van Ermengem). When dried they may retain their vitality for as long as a year.

Its most characteristic property is the production of a very powerful toxin. According to Van Ermengem considerable differences are met with in the virulence of the toxins produced in the different strains isolated. Toxin production is much more uniform when glucose is present in the nutrient culture medium. The bacillus (like *B. tetani*) will not grow to any extent in the animal body, but produces its poisonous effects by the toxins which it excretes into the nutrient material in which it is growing—a true exotoxin. When introduced into suitable animals (rabbits, monkeys, cats, pigeons, etc.) either by subcutaneous, intraperitoneal or intravenous injection or by feeding, the toxin reproduces in a very definite way the characteristic symptoms of botulism. As little as 0·0003 to 0·001 c.c. of a broth culture may kill a rabbit. In every case the symptoms only come on after an incubation period which usually is not less than twenty-four hours. The most characteristic symptoms by inoculation are produced with cats.

It is rather characteristic that the symptoms can be readily reproduced by feeding, although of course considerably larger doses are required. Monkeys, guinea-pigs and mice are the most suitable for these feeding experiments. Small monkeys (*Rhesus*), for example, are killed in from 24–34 hours, with all the symptoms of the condition, after feeding with small quantities of toxin. Cats are very resistant to feeding and enormous doses must be given. On the other hand large numbers of the bacilli, apart from their toxin, can be fed to rabbits or guinea-pigs without causing poisoning symptoms, the organism being unable to produce its toxin in the animal body.

The toxin is not highly resistant and is rapidly destroyed by heating to 70–80° C.

Dickson (1917 a) noted that during the investigation of several outbreaks a number of fowls became ill with paralysis, etc., and died after eating food which had caused the human outbreaks. B. botulinus was isolated from the food in the crop and gizzard.

The pathological anatomy lesions in inoculated animals have been worked out with great care. Marinesco, and later, Kempner and Pollack, also Römer and Stein found early degeneration changes in the spinal grey matter, chiefly of the anterior horns, and in the medulla oblongata, while Van Ermengem found degeneration in the nuclei of the ocular nerves, the hypoglossal and the vagus. Cloudy and fatty degeneration of the cells of the liver, kidneys, and other organs also occur. Lesions of the cells of the cerebrum do not occur.

According to Kempner and Schepilewski the toxin has a special affinity for cerebro-spinal tissue and is fixed and neutralized by admixture with brain substance.

The methods and paths of infection have not been so satisfactorily demonstrated as the pathological nature of the condition. Outbreaks have most frequently followed the consumption of liver, blood and other varieties of sausage and also after eating ham, but have also been met with in connection with smoked meat, tinned meat, stuffed geese, raw and salted fish and from the use of certain non-meat foods, such as preserved beans. The majority of the recent American cases have been traced to home-canned vegetables or fruit. Cases with somewhat similar symptoms, but without bacteriological confirmation have been described after the consumption of crab and of oysters. In but few of these outbreaks has B. botulinus been isolated and the diagnosis rests upon the clinical picture.

In the Ellezelles outbreak from which Van Ermengem (1897) first isolated *B. botulinus*, the ham was derived from a healthy animal, the rest of which was consumed without harm. The affected ham had been laid at the bottom of the pickling cask and covered with the pickling solution, while the other ham from the same animal, which was quite harmless, was laid above it and not covered by the liquid. The poisonous ham was not putrid but had a strong rancid odour.

Römer (1900) isolated the bacillus from a ham pickled in brine which caused four cases of botulism, the rest of the animal being eaten without symptoms. The pig was killed two months before the outbreak and the ham was noticed to smell badly after being dried. Evidently only part of the ham itself was affected since others ate of it without symptoms, but only those parts which were normal in appearance and smell. The affected portions were blue-grey in colour with a rancid butyric acid odour and contained long, sporing bacilli. The normal parts showed no bacilli.

The outbreak at Darmstadt in 1904 described by Fischer (1906) is a good example of an outbreak not of meat origin and illustrates the high fatality often met with, since eleven died out of twenty-one attacked. The cases occurred at a cookery school and followed the consumption of a bean salad prepared and canned three months previously by one of the cooks at the school. The salad was eaten by twenty-four persons. The beans had a rancid odour when the can was opened, especially noticeable after the addition of the vinegar. They were not cooked but merely rinsed and warmed before being eaten. A bacillus almost identical with *B. botulinus* was isolated and yielded a toxin fatal to guinea-pigs in doses of 0·0003 c.c. The remainder of the uncooked salad filtered through a Berkefeld filter was very toxic to mice and other animals.

Van Ermengem gives two other instances in which *B. botulinus* was isolated. One at Orö (Denmark) in 1901, affecting three persons, one with fatal result, and due to the consumption of mackerel preserved in vinegar. The fish examined some weeks later had a pronounced butyric acid smell.

The other was at Iseghem in West Flanders in 1906, affected eight out of twelve persons in one family, and was due to eating a ham which showed no abnormal taste or smell.

This bacillus was also isolated by Ornstein (1913) from an infected ham which caused two cases, while the bacillus was also isolated from the spleen of one of the fatal cases.

Another outbreak from ham in which B. botulinus was isolated was reported by Schumacher (1913) in which six members of one family were taken ill after eating raw ham. The four children recovered but the father and mother died. The bacillus was isolated both from the ham and from the spleen of one of the fatal cases. Wilbur and Ophüls (1914) describe an interesting outbreak in America in November, 1913, of twelve cases of illness with one fatal case, which presented the symptoms of botulism and which was due to canned string beans served without preliminary heating. The beans were canned by one of the party the summer before. B. botulinus was not isolated but none of the beans from the tin actually used were available for examination. Nothing abnormal about the beans was noted at the time.

As a rule no evidences of putrefactive changes were noticeable in the poisonous food, but Schede (1916) in a recent outbreak of three cases in June, 1916, at Charlottenburg, with two deaths, due to eating ham obtained from a pig killed the previous autumn, reports that the ham was obviously not good when eaten, so much so that the remainder with the bone was thrown away at the time.

Considerable diversity of opinion exists as to the prevalence of this peculiar type of food poisoning and as to its specific identity. As mentioned above no authentic outbreaks appear to have occurred in this country. On the other hand Dorendorf (1917) in a recent lecture on this subject in Germany considers that isolated cases or small groups may be not infrequent. He records that over a period of three months he saw in a Military Hospital in East Germany seven cases of botulism, five being sporadic cases and the other two in one group. In no instance, however, was the diagnosis confirmed bacteriologically, while this is not a disease which one would expect to occur as sporadic cases.

Dickson (1917 b) in America considers that the disease is more common than is shown by the records. He states that in an investigation of unrecorded cases of food poisoning which occurred on the Pacific Coast of the United States during the previous six years he located eleven outbreaks of botulism in which twenty-nine persons were ill and twenty-three died. From three of these he states that he established the diagnosis of botulism by the isolation of B. botulinus from the affected food. In this paper Dickson tabulates these and a further eleven outbreaks in the Western States of America, eighteen being on the Pacific coast—seventeen in California and one in Oregon State. In all eighty-one persons were ill and sixty-five died, a mortality of 68 per cent. In eighteen outbreaks in which the source of the poisoning was recognized eleven were of vegetable origin (six home-canned string beans, and one each from other fruits or vegetables), two to bottled clam broth and the other five to different meat foods.

The most definite fact which emerges from a consideration of these and other outbreaks is that in none of them were the implicated foods eaten in the fresh state, the toxic properties only developing after the food had been stored. Not only had the food been kept for a long time but usually had been preserved under conditions which were obviously unsatis- factory, such as insufficient pickling, defective smoking, inadequate canning, etc., while it had then been eaten without being cooked. It is quite evident that the develop- ment of poisonous properties is due to an invasion of other- wise healthy food by B. botulinus from outside sources and this can only occur when suitable anaerobic conditions are provided. This bacillus must be considered, as Van Ermen- gem insists, as a pathogenic saprophyte.

Dickson (1915), in an experimental study, infected cans of string beans and other vegetables with B. botulinus and kept the inoculated cans at room temperatures for three to twelve months. Of twelve cases so infected four were rejected as the control tests were unsatisfactory, while B. botulinus was isolated in pure culture from six of the remaining eight tins.

Dickson (1917 *b*) tested the efficiency of the so-called cold-pack method of canning vegetables to kill *B. botulinus*. This is a method much recommended for home canning and consists of heating the filled jars at the temperature of boiling water. He found this method quite inefficient to kill *B. botulinus* spores when these were experimentally added to jars of peas, beans and corn, and subsequently heated for 120 to 180 minutes.

As regards the conditions under which it is found in nature and the paths of infection to the food our knowledge is of the scantiest. Van Ermengem was unable to find this bacillus in fifty-two different samples examined by him, consisting of the excreta of domestic animals (pig, cow, horse, duck, fowl), intestinal content of different kinds of fishes, soil, mud, manure, etc.

The only positive finding which appears to be recorded is that of Kempner and Pollack, who isolated a bacillus from the excreta of a pig in Berlin which they identified with *B. botulinus*. Van Ermengem examined this strain and found that it closely resembled his pathogenic bacillus from the Ellezelles outbreak but culturally was most like the Darmstadt bacillus. Kempner obtained an antitoxin serum by injecting it into animals and this serum was capable of neutralizing the toxins both of the Ellezelles and of the Darmstadt bacilli.

More exact knowledge as to the distribution of this organism in nature is very desirable.

The prevention of the conditions favourable to the infection and growth of *B. botulinus* should not be difficult. Sausages and other forms of prepared food must be manufactured from good and clean materials only and the methods of preservation must be satisfactory and efficient. Unlike toxins of the Gaertner group efficient cooking destroys the toxins of *B. botulinus*, so it is important that all such foods should be properly cooked, either in course of manufacture or before being eaten. Foods of this character which exhibit a butyric acid-like smell should be particularly regarded with suspicion. Van Ermengem also recommends that in salting the brine should contain at least 10 per cent. sodium chloride, since *B. botulinus* will not grow in media containing more than 6 per cent. sodium chloride.

Note. During the spring and early summer of 1918 a number of cases of illness occurred which clinically somewhat resembled those met with in outbreaks of botulism. Several observers suggested that they were cases of botulism, and such an attractive label obtained wide credence in the daily press and to a limited extent in medical papers. The cases mostly occurred between February and June and were met with in London, Sheffield, Birmingham and other large towns with a few single or groups of cases in other areas. A careful analysis of the symptoms by anyone cognizant of the classical features of botulism would have shown that the differences from that condition were more noticeable than the resemblances, a knowledge of the mode of causation of botulism would at once have thrown suspicion upon such a diagnosis, while a careful study of the epidemiological aspect would have been sufficient to remove any grounds for assuming any relationship to this variety of food poisoning. Indeed as soon as the trained investigator, apart from the clinician, took up the matter it was evident that the diagnosis of botulism rested upon no scientific foundation, and some non-committal title such as Polioencephalitis was a more fitting designation for the cases. *B. botulinus* was searched for, but naturally never isolated.

See Memorandum by Local Government Board, *Brit. Med. Journ.* 1918, May 18th, 573; G. H. Melland, *Brit. Med. Journ.* 1918, May 18th, 559, and May 25th, 587; W. Benton, *Public Health*, 1918, XXXI. 111; W. G. Savage, *Public Health*, 1918, XXXI, 112, etc.

REFERENCES.

E. C. Dickson (1915). *Journ. Am. Med. Assoc.* LXV. 492.
—— (1917 a). *Journ. Am. Vet. Med. Assoc.* L. 612.
—— (1917 b). *Journ. Am. Med. Assoc.* LXVII 966.
—— (1918). *Botulism.* Monograph of the Rockfeller Institute of Medical Research. New York.
Dorendorf (1917). *Deut. med. Woch.* XLIII. 1531 and 1554.
Fischer (1906). *Zeitschr. f. klin. Medicin*, LIX. 58.
Kempner and Pollack (1897). *Deut. med. Woch.* XXIII. 505.
—— and Schepilewski (1898). *Zeit. f. Hyg.* XXVII. 213.
Marinesco (1897). *Presse médicale*, V. 41.
McIntosh (1917). *Medical Research Com. Special Reports*, No. 12.
Ornstein (1913). *Zeit. Chemotherap.* I. 458.
Römer (1900). *Centralb. f. Bakt.* Orig. XXVII. 857.
—— and Stein (1904). *Arch. f. Ophthalmologie*, LVIII. 291.
Schede (1916). *Medizinische Klinik*, XII. 1309.
Schumacher (1913). *Münch. med. Woch.* LX. 125.
T. Stephenson (1892). *Brit. Med. Journ.* II. 1326.
Van Ermengem (1897). *Zeit. f. Hyg.* XXVI. 1.
—— (1912). Kolle und Wassermann, *Handbuch der Pathogenen Microorganismen*, IV. 909.
Wilbur and Ophüls (1914). *Arch. of Int. Med.* XIV. 589.

CHAPTER X

SOURCES AND METHODS OF INFECTION IN FOOD POISONING OUTBREAKS

THE data given in earlier chapters make it evident that as bacteriological investigations of outbreaks become more exact and complete, Gaertner group bacilli are isolated in an increased proportion of instances, and while it is possible that individual cases and limited outbreaks of illness may be due to putrefactive changes in the food consumed, it may be accepted generally that infection of food with bacilli of the Gaertner group must be looked upon as the usual cause of outbreaks of food poisoning of bacterial origin.

In instances of poisoning of the nature of putrefactive intoxication, if there are any such cases, it is not necessary to trace back the matter further since there is no question of specific infection with a definite bacterium, the toxic condition of the meat being produced by the growth of bacteria which are widely present in nature as saprophytes.

When, however, we are dealing with infection of the food with specific bacilli it becomes necessary to carry the matter a stage further and to inquire how the food became infected with these particular bacilli and from whence they were derived.

It is unfortunate that so many of the British recorded outbreaks are lacking in information in regard to the paths of infection. Many of the recorders of these outbreaks seem to have deemed it sufficient to prove the possibility of excretal contamination of the food material in question, and having done so appear to have regarded this as a sufficient explanation of the whole occurrence.

In a large proportion of the outbreaks no attempt seems to have been made to get at the actual sources of infection, and this applies to the large as well as to the small outbreaks. There are many lacunae in our knowledge which it is most desirable to fill up. A few, however, of the records contain

information of the highest value, while many of the continental recorded outbreaks have been more carefully worked
out from this point of view.

It cannot be too strongly emphasised that outbreaks of
bacterial food poisoning are due to *specific* infection and not
to general infection of the food with ordinary excretal bacilli,
and therefore no inquiry into an outbreak can have any claim
to completeness unless the source of this specific infection has
been traced or at least carefully sought for.

In connection with such inquiries two important possibilities require careful consideration.

Evidence as to disease in the animals supplying the food affected.

The evidence as to the health of the animals supplying
the meat in the reports dealing with individual outbreaks in
this country is very meagre, the majority making no mention
of it. In a few cases the investigator states that he was in-
formed that the animals were healthy, but as this is usually
the evidence of highly interested persons it is not very
valuable.

In only two of the British outbreaks recorded in the
writer's report to the Local Government Board (Savage,
1913) was any evidence given that the animal was diseased.
In one, the Murrow outbreak, amongst the bones, etc., used
to make the brawn was a pig's foot which was obviously
diseased and which from the description available had an
abscess on it. The pig was sufficiently affected to have to
be carted to the place of slaughter.

In the Limerick outbreak (McWeeney, 1909) the available
evidence is not very precise, but the meat was purchased
ready killed by the contractor and at *an unusually low price.*
No reliable information was obtainable as to the condition
of the animal prior to or at the time of slaughter, but since
the butcher who sold it to the contractor would appear to
have sold it below cost price it is highly probable that it
was not sound healthy meat.

In striking contrast are the continental records. Of forty

outbreaks tabulated in the above Government Report, in 50 per cent. it was reported that the meat was derived from a diseased animal. The diseased conditions found were gastro-enteritis, etc. eight, udder disease two, puerperal sepsis one, local abscesses three, other diseases six.

The discrepancy between these two sets of records is partly to be accounted for by the better system of meat inspection in Germany and Belgium, where most of these continental outbreaks occurred, thus allowing diseased conditions in the animals to be more readily traced, partly to a more general recognition abroad of the association of these outbreaks with diseased animals (the condition not being inquired into for many of the English outbreaks) and to some extent to the fact that the continental series were mainly large well-defined outbreaks easier to investigate.

Evidence of disease in the animals supplying the affected food is best illustrated in connection with the outbreaks spread by milk. The nine outbreaks of milk origin mentioned in Table I merit individual consideration.

For four of them (Greenwich, Aberdeen, Edinburgh and the first Newcastle-under-Lyme outbreak) no detailed investigations were made, or at least recorded, in regard to the condition of the animals supplying the milk.

In the 1894 Manchester outbreak, involving 160 cases, it was found that a cow affected with an inflamed udder (mastitis) had been removed from the farm supplying the incriminated milk two days after the outbreak and was killed two days later. No bacteriological examination was made of this cow so that full proof of the association was not obtained but a Gaertner bacillus was isolated from the mixed milk.

In the Bakewell outbreak (1908) all the infected milk was traced back to a farm upon which a cow had calved five days before the cases developed, and the milk of which was added to the implicated supply two days previous to the outbreak. No bacteriological investigations or examination of the cow were made.

The extensive outbreak at Newcastle-upon-Tyne (Kerr and Hutchens, 1914) in 1913, involving at least 523 persons, was spread by milk derived from a cow which had recently calved and which then had been added to the herd and her milk mixed with the rest. The cow had shown signs of illness a day or two before and died almost coincidently with the occurrence of the first cases of the outbreak. *B. enteritidis* was isolated from the internal organs of this cow, from milk obtained from the udder after death, as well as from the stools of seven of the persons attacked.

The Withnell and Chorley outbreak (Sergeant, 1914) affected 317 persons and was due to *B. enteritidis* conveyed in milk and derived from a cow which suffered from ill-defined illness, with (apparently) udder inflammation, for several days before the outbreak and died the day on which the first cases developed.

The facts elicited in the outbreak in 1914 at Newcastle-under-Lyme are of particular interest. 468 cases were recorded with two deaths. The milk was obtained through two vendors, but all came from one farm. Inquiries at this farm elicited that a cow had been purchased from a dealer while in calf, about four weeks prior to the outbreak. Some two weeks later (i.e. about two weeks before the outbreak) she calved at the farm and two days later fell ill with what was believed to be "milk fever." Abscesses, which had to be opened, developed in one leg. Notwithstanding this condition the milk of this animal continued to be mixed with the rest and was sold up to four days before the outbreak, when it was withheld owing to the purulent nature of the discharge from the abscesses. The milk was then given instead to four calves all of which fell ill and two died.

The blood of this cow completely agglutinated *B. enteritidis*, isolated from the organs of one of the fatal cases, proving that it had been infected with that organism. Subsequent examination of the discharges of this cow showed the presence of *B. enteritidis* in the urine and uterine discharges. The milk of this diseased animal was examined by Delépine on a number of occasions after the outbreak but at first without finding *B. enteritidis*. The milk then had a normal appearance, but two further samples examined fifty and seventy-eight days respectively after the beginning of the

outbreak showed evidence of mastitis and from one of them
B. enteritidis was isolated.

In the outbreak in Giessen in October, 1891, described by
Gaffky (1892), the vehicle was milk derived from a herd
amongst which was a cow which had suffered from a local
inflammatory swelling on the shoulder and also from
diarrhoea.

The isolation of *B. enteritidis* from cases of acute mastitis
in cows is discussed on p. 83.

In view of the fact that it is sometimes accepted that the
flesh of swine fever animals is harmless to man the following
outbreak described by Müller (1918) is of great interest as
showing that *B. suipestifer* from pigs suffering from swine
fever can originate outbreaks of human food poisoning under
favourable circumstances. In this case these were the consumption of the bacilli in livers which were not cooked. The
outbreak also shows the great protection afforded by cooking.

In February, 1917, seven pigs fell ill and were slaughtered.
Six of them were markedly ill and when examined after
death showed haemorrhagic necrotic areas in the lungs
indicative of pleuro-pneumonia, but with only slight changes
in the intestines. They were diagnosed as suffering from
Schweineseuche and Schweinepest. The veterinary inspector
condemned the intestines, lungs and spleen as unfit, but the
rest of the organs and the carcases were passed for food.
The seventh pig showed only trifling signs of illness when
alive and no signs of disease when killed. The flesh of this
animal was used at the farm itself, being first cooked, then
chopped up and made into sausage meat. To this chopped-
up sausage meat was added the livers (all free from naked-
eye evidence of disease) of all the seven pigs. Before this
meat was filled into skins and recooked as sausages part of
it was eaten by five persons. Two ate scarcely any of it and
remained well but the other three all became ill with fever,
diarrhoea, headache and vomiting, the symptoms lasting
three to six days. All recovered.

All the persons who ate the sausage meat after it was filled
into skins and recooked remained unaffected.

Part of the sausage meat and livers, however, owing to lack

of casings, could not be so used. It remained over until next day and was then eaten by fifteen persons all of whom became ill. The symptoms were as above, but some were more severe and they lasted from six to eight days. All ultimately recovered. From this sausage meat *B. suipestifer* was isolated.

The flesh of the six animals was consumed without harm. Illness therefore only resulted when the livers of these pigs were eaten in an uncooked condition. That these animals were suffering from swine fever is further shown by the fact that on the same premises, some before, some subsequently, eleven other pigs died and examination showed that their lungs, livers, spleens and kidneys were strongly infected with *B. suipestifer*.

Evidence pointing to infection of the food subsequent to slaughter.

A study of recorded outbreaks in this country shows, in a considerable number of them, that infection of the foodstuff may with great probability be accepted as taking place during or after preparation of the animal for sale.

The evidence is cumulative rather than conclusive in particular outbreaks. The following general summary will be sufficient to demonstrate its nature.

(a) *In many of the recorded outbreaks while no information was available showing that the animal was diseased, clear evidence was forthcoming that during preparation for sale extensive excretal contamination was possible and likely.* In outbreak after outbreak abundant possibilities of such contamination have been shown to exist although as explained elsewhere this argument is of limited validity.

Three examples out of many may be mentioned to illustrate the abundant opportunities for excretal contamination.

In the Mansfield outbreak (No. 18) the potted meat, the consumption of which caused the outbreak, was put to set and cool in the preparing-room, which was used for slaughtering the pigs. Pigs had been slaughtered there the day before the incriminated food was made. Further, the utensils used for preparing the potted meat were used equally in connection with the slaughtering. The bowl used for ladling the gravy of the potted meat was, for example, used in dressing the carcases.

In the Bacup (No. 84) outbreak the vehicle of infection was roast leg of pork. The legs were stuffed, roasted and sold as boneless legs of pork, so that considerable manipulation was required. The other parts of the pigs caused no illness, and, as it was the legs which were infected, it is reasonable to assume that infection was post-slaughter. An obvious means of possible contamination was found, since it was ascertained that the man who prepared the legs for roasting and removed the bones was also engaged in slaughtering and in *gut cleaning*.

In the Trowbridge outbreak (No. 109) due to infected chitterlings (i.e. the large intestine and stomach of the pig), the following was the method of preparation at the time of the outbreak. The guts, divided into lengths, were placed in a wooden tub containing warm water. Then piece by piece the lengths were taken out, their contents emptied into a bowl, by pressure between the thumb and finger, and each piece replaced in the same tub. Fresh water was then placed in the tub and the pieces washed in it, no running water being used. The pieces of gut were then placed in a lead lined trough filled with brine, said to be in the proportion of $1\frac{1}{4}$ cwt. salt to thirty gallons of water. The chitterlings remain in the brine for a varying length of time, being removed as customers send for supplies. The premises were old and there was a general lack of cleanliness.

It is obvious that under such conditions one section of infected gut would have ample opportunity to contaminate other batches, while the methods used would not remove all the excretal contents. No recognized period for brining was employed, this varying with the demand. The infected chitterlings were in the brine for from thirty minutes to six hours, but, from the facts obtained, could not have been there longer.

(b) *In many cases the meat during preparation was so treated, e.g. by boiling or other form of cooking, that any bacilli or toxins in it must inevitably have been destroyed, and that since the meat was shown to contain Gaertner group bacilli they must have been added after the preparation stages were completed.*

This argument is particularly applicable in the case of brawn and some other prepared foods, and must be considered of great weight. The fact that the food has undergone preparation even involving heating cannot, however, be taken as conclusive in itself that the infection was post-slaughter. Trade expressions frequently will not bear scientific interpretations, and boiling to the meat purveyor may not mean a temperature of anything like 100° C., either at any time or over a prolonged period. The low temperatures reached in ordinary cooking have already been considered.

Also there are sometimes opportunities for re-infection from the same source after cooking, e.g. from infected utensils, vessels, etc. In the Trowbridge outbreak, for example, the cooked chitterlings were put in cold water in the same bath in which they were put to soak before the boiling.

(c) *In a number of cases the specific food which caused the outbreak was non-infectious (or at least did not cause infection) at first and only became so after the lapse of a definite period of time.*

The following outbreak at Cressage in 1900 is a good example.

At a farmhouse three geese were killed and a certain widow helped to prepare and cook them. The giblets were stewed September 26th and eaten by the farmhouse people, while the geese were cooked and eaten the next day (September 27th). Both lots of food were eaten without harm. On September 27th about 2 p.m. the widow took home a portion of the giblets (consisting of gizzard and other parts), the giblets gravy, pieces of goose and slices of beef. These were placed in her pantry at home and eaten cold for supper the same evening without being recooked. After the consumption of this meat seven persons were ill and two died. Twenty-seven hours elapsed between the cooking of the giblets and their consumption.

A similar latency of infection is observable in a number of

other outbreaks. While this point is important by itself it is quite insufficient to prove that infection took place between the date when the meat was non-infective and when it was infective, since infection is to some extent a question of dosage.

Even in the Cressage case, which is of great interest, it by no means follows that infection was subsequent to cooking. The geese may have been diseased and the first cooking sufficient to kill nearly all the Gaertner bacilli, but not quite all, a few surviving. The twenty-seven hours in the warm weather would have given them abundant opportunities to multiply in the rich nutrient material, and so render this food highly infective.

This argument is therefore of value, but is not conclusive in itself.

(d) *A further point is that since other portions of the animal were eaten without harm the animal itself could not have been diseased, and the cause of the outbreak: inferentially, therefore, the food infection must have been after death.*

This argument is adopted in many of the English reports, and while it is not without weight, it is only very partially true. It implies that Gaertner group infections of the food-supplying animals are generalised infections, and that the bacilli are present in all the organs and parts of the body. This would seem not to be the case, and localised lesions, such as the leg lesion in the Murrow pig, would appear to occur. In the Limerick and Murrow outbreaks, in which disease of the animal was highly probable, the other parts of the animals were eaten without apparent harm.

In many of the continental outbreaks the animals supplying the food were definitely diseased, but while the meat of certain parts of the animal caused food poisoning, consumption of the rest of the flesh was without apparent harm.

The question is probably not merely one of a local versus a general infection, but also one of dosage, the bacilli being more distributed in certain parts of the body, while the cooking processes to which different parts are subjected are not equal.

(e) *A large proportion of the outbreaks has been associated*

with foodstuffs which are very liable to bacterial contamination,
and which when so contaminated allow marked multiplication
of the added bacteria.

This is an argument of great importance and weight. The
prevalence of brawn and pork pies as vehicles of infection
has already been discussed. Both contain a good deal of
jelly and are admirable nutrient media for bacteria, while
both cool slowly and in so doing afford, over a long period, a
temperature suitable for very rapid multiplication of Gaertner or other bacilli. While brawn is not invariably sterilized
during its preparation it is so in most cases, and as such
provides a medium artificially sterilized and freed from competing bacilli, a third factor favouring rapid multiplication.
The frequency with which foods containing an excess of
gelatinous matter have served as the vehicle in food poisoning
outbreaks was first drawn attention to by Ballard in his
classical report to the Local Government Board in 1890.

A further point in connection with these made-foods is
the frequency with which these articles have to be handled,
thus increasing the liability to infection.

(*f*) *In a certain proportion of the outbreaks the vehicle of*
infection is not of animal nature at all. For these it is obvious
that infection of the food during or subsequent to preparation must have taken place. The following outbreak at
Clapham in 1911 is a good example.

Tinned pineapple was purchased on the Saturday, opened
on Sunday and made into a jelly by the cook on Sunday
morning. It was then kept in the larder for about nine
hours when it was placed on the table and eaten at 9 p.m. by
eight persons, all of whom were taken ill and one died. There
was a definite incubation period and the severity of the
symptoms were not in proportion to the dose, so that it was
clearly not a case of metallic poisoning.

No bacteriological investigations were made, but this outbreak was probably due to Gaertner or other bacilli which
had infected the jelly and multiplied abundantly in it during
the nine hours the food was kept in the larder on a hot July
day in 1911. The jelly also would have been hot to start
with.

The presence of a material (jelly) capable of serving as a nutrient medium for the bacteria is here the important thing. The report gives no clue as to how the jelly could have become infected.

While no one of the considerations mentioned as evidence of infection subsequent to the death of the animal is, in itself, sufficient to prove the point, they are each of value, and their cumulative evidence is in many cases quite sufficient to prove that the bacteria obtained access to the food after slaughter.

There is one important argument on the other side which has not been mentioned. It is only in extremely rare cases that the sheep has been the animal furnishing the meat which has served as the vehicle of infection. It may be advanced that if post-slaughter infection were common we should meet with many more such cases, since we know that Gaertner group bacilli inoculated upon mutton will multiply abundantly. The probable explanation is the comparative infrequency with which mutton is used in the preparation of made foods. It is chiefly eaten in the form of roast or boiled meat, and the joints being small are more likely to be efficiently cooked. There are no known diseases of the sheep due to Gaertner group bacilli.

Sources of infection.

The considerations just discussed show that while in a certain number of instances the source of infection is straightforward, the vehicle of infection being meat or milk derived from an animal suffering from disease (general or localized) caused by one or other member of the Gaertner group of bacteria, in the remaining outbreaks (and this probably constitutes a considerable majority) there is no evidence of such a causal connection, while in at least some cases it is manifestly untrue, the vehicle of infection not being derived from an animal at all. If we are to attain to reliable preventive measures it is essential to endeavour to trace out and ascertain the sources of infection in all cases, and especially for those in which Gaertner group bacilli have gained access from outside the food itself. There are three separate hypotheses which may be advanced and which require detailed consideration.

Hypothesis A. That the Gaertner group bacilli which are the cause of the food poisoning outbreaks are of human origin, the meat being infected with pathogenic Gaertner bacilli from a human source, i.e. a case of disease (paratyphoid fever) or a carrier case.

This view has been advanced by Conradi and by Rommeler. It has in its favour the fact that paratyphoid bacilli carriers have been proved to exist and that by analogy with typhoid carriers such carriers are potential, and may be actual, sources of infection.

It may be accepted as demonstrated that outbreaks of paratyphoid fever, like outbreaks of typhoid fever, are frequently spread by carriers, but this is a very different proposition to suggesting that attacks of food poisoning can be originated by paratyphoid fever carriers. As far as we know *B. paratyphosus B* carriers always set up outbreaks of paratyphoid fever.

An interesting outbreak of this kind is that recorded by Sacquépée and Bellot (1910). The outbreak of paratyphoid fever was caused by food, and the evidence suggests that this was infected by an assistant cook who had suffered from an ill-defined illness a short time previously. Paratyphoid bacilli were isolated from his excreta but only some months after the outbreak. The possibility of these bacilli being derived from a slight attack at the time of the outbreak was not fully excluded by the investigators, nor was the real nature of his ill-defined illness bacteriologically ascertained.

Trautmann has advanced the hypothesis that in meat poisoning outbreaks we have to deal chiefly with an intoxication from ingested toxins, while in paratyphoid fever with an infection with a few of the same bacilli (paratyphoid bacilli), which only cause disease symptoms after a definite incubation period.

If this hypothesis were true, in most outbreaks some cases would be acute with the ordinary food poisoning symptoms, while others would be cases of paratyphoid fever.

This is by no means the case, although, as explained on p. 48, a few protracted cases of infection are met with.

It has been pointed out that in several outbreaks the meat, when undoubtedly infected with Gaertner group bacilli, was eaten on the first day without harm or with only a small percentage of attacks, although very toxic on the second and subsequent days. On this hypothesis, at least, some of the persons who ate the meat on the first day should have developed paratyphoid fever. There is no evidence of a single such case in these outbreaks.

We have evidence that *B. paratyphosus B* can cause acute gastro-enteritis, simulating a food poisoning outbreak, in the very interesting outbreak recorded by Bainbridge and Dudfield (1911). They record a number of cases of acute gastro-enteritis in which the onset and symptoms were indistinguishable from those met with in ordinary food poisoning outbreaks, and in which *B. paratyphosus B* was the organism found. Careful investigation failed to find any article of food which could be shown to be the vehicle of infection while a number of the cases occurred in different places and on different dates. The cases were connected, but it was one of contact, not a common food supply. In this outbreak the evidence was in favour of a human source of infection.

McWeeney (1916) records the case of a man who was admitted to a Dublin hospital suffering from marked collapse and other symptoms. *B. aertrycke* was isolated. It is not clear if this was a case of food poisoning associated with food, or was a case comparable to those of Bainbridge and Dudfield.

According to the writer's view (in contradistinction to the view accepted widely in Germany that *B. paratyphosus B* and *B. suipestifer* are identical) no food poisoning outbreaks have been shown to be due to *B. paratyphosus B* but all to *B. aertrycke* (*vel B. suipestifer*) or *B. enteritidis*, with possibly a few closely allied forms. To accept the carrier view we have therefore to postulate that human beings can and do act as carriers of *B. enteritidis* or *B. aertrycke*. Only a very few such cases have been recorded.

That *B. aertrycke*, like *B. paratyphosus B*, can persist after

infection through food poisoning in the human intestine is
shown by investigations in connection with a very extensive
outbreak amongst troops in France in April 1918, involving
over 1000 cases. The outbreak could not be traced to the consumption of any one article of food but from the evidence
it was highly probable that it was due to food infection.
The cases, however, did not develop explosively but extended
over several weeks, most of the cases occurring within a
period of ten days. Perry and Tidy (1919), who describe the
outbreak, considered that the primary infection was due to a
human carrier, although no convincing evidence is adduced,
and that the secondary cases which were common were due
to the same cause. The outbreak was definitely traced to
B. aertrycke, its exact place in the group being worked out
by agglutination and absorption tests, while this bacillus
was isolated from many of the cases and identified as the
cause by agglutination tests with the blood of cases. Perry
and Tidy made some valuable observations upon the persistence of these bacilli in the excreta of cases, studying forty-
four cases for this purpose. In the early stages in many cases
B. aertrycke was present in practically a pure culture. They
found that 50 per cent. had ceased to excrete this organism
by the end of the fourth week, while at the end of the seventh
week only two were positive. One continued positive for
fourteen weeks and the bacilli were still present at the time
of the report.

The only outbreaks in this country definitely ascribed to
a human carrier are those at Wrexham (1910) and at Brighton (1917). The Wrexham evidence is inconclusive. The
cook to whom is ascribed the rôle of carrier is said not to
have eaten any of the incriminated pie, and her blood
reacted to the Gaertner group bacillus isolated as the cause
of the outbreak in one out of four tests. From her faeces
after the outbreak members of the Gaertner group were
isolated, but no evidence is advanced that they were identical
with the Wrexham bacillus. The cook might have been
slightly infected without showing any obtrusive symptoms.

In the Brighton outbreak, investigated by Forbes and the
writer (Savage and Forbes, 1918), twenty-eight cases of food

poisoning in a general hospital were traced to the consumption of fried fish. The evidence showed that the fish was infected in the hospital and the rest of it was eaten in the town without any evidence of ill-health. The serum of the kitchen maid, who had abundant opportunities for contaminating the fish, since she sliced, floured and cooked it, showed well-marked Gaertner group agglutinins. From the internal organs of a fatal case and from the excreta of this kitchen maid a highly pathogenic bacillus was isolated, which while serologically identical with *B. enteritidis* showed at first cultural deviations (i.e. diminished fermentation properties). The existence of these differences proved the absolute identity of the two bacilli. Very detailed inquiries were made which showed that the kitchen maid disliked fish and had not eaten any of the infected fish and that she had not suffered in the slightest degree at the time of the outbreak or showed any symptoms of illness. The investigators concluded that she was a carrier of this bacillus and had infected the fish and caused the outbreak. There was no available evidence as to how this girl became infected and a carrier.

In a number of outbreaks the carrier hypothesis is suggested as the source of infection (for example, Bernstein and Fish, 1916), but as a rule it is a suggestion only and there is no actual evidence to support the contention.

While therefore there appears to be a probability that a certain number of outbreaks may be ascribed to infection of the food from a human carrier, the existing evidence suggests that such cases are few in number. Evidence is lacking as to the persistence of these bacilli in the human intestine after outbreaks of food poisoning, although from analogy with animals it is likely that in some cases they may persist for long periods.

The human carrier hypothesis cannot be advanced as a general explanation for all or even for most outbreaks, while this view does not explain the proved association of many outbreaks with the consumption of the flesh of diseased animals.

Hypothesis B. That the Gaertner group bacilli which set up

*the food poisoning outbreaks are derived from ordinary faecal
infection of the food.*

The acceptance of this view, of course, implies that the
true Gaertner group bacilli are *natural* intestinal inhabitants.
In view of this hypothesis this question was considered in
considerable detail in Chapter VI. It was there shown that
true Gaertner group bacilli cannot be considered as natural
inhabitants of the animal intestine.

The writer from his own and recorded investigations be-
lieves this hypothesis, which is so frequently given in reports
upon food poisoning outbreaks as a sufficient explanation,
is without foundation, and that any support which it has
received from bacteriological findings is due to insufficient
cultural and agglutinative differentiation of the bacilli isolated.

Also strongly against this view is the fact that present day
methods for the preparation of meat for sale frequently
allow great possibilities of contamination with excremen-
titious matters. This contamination is especially liable to
occur with made-foods, such as sausages, brawn and meat
pies. The two former often show the presence of enormous
numbers of faecal bacilli.

The writer has also shown that when flesh, brawn, etc., are
inoculated with Gaertner bacilli and with *B. coli* both
multiply very rapidly, so that there is no reason for assuming
that under natural conditions any Gaertner group bacilli
which gained access to meat would be overgrown by concomitant *B. coli*, thus preventing infection.

This being the case, if simple faecal contamination is a
sufficient explanation, food poisoning outbreaks should be
extremely common instead of comparatively rare.

The available data conclusively disproves the correctness
of this hypothesis.

*Hypothesis C. That food poisoning outbreaks are due to
infection of the food with virulent Gaertner group organisms
(or other special bacilli) derived from animals which are either
at the time suffering from disease due to Gaertner group bacilli
or acting as carriers of these bacilli.*

This is the view which the writer has advanced as the one

which best explains all or most of the phenomena of food poisoning due to Gaertner group bacilli.

This hypothesis is adequate to explain the outbreaks associated with the consumption of the meat of a diseased animal, and is also capable of explaining the outbreaks in which infection occurs during or after preparation of the food.

As set out in Chapter VI there is a considerable number of animal diseases due to Gaertner group bacilli. Many of them affect animals used for human food, others animals (rats and mice) which have opportunities of infecting human food.

While true Gaertner group bacilli are not natural inhabitants of the healthy animal intestine, they are very occasionally found to be present in it and in a few cases have been found in made-foods, such as sausages. Their occurrence, which is rare, is probably due to the presence of carrier bacilli in animals recovering from infection from a Gaertner group organism.

Zwick and Weichel examined 177 mice and in twenty-eight found they were acting as carriers of Gaertner group bacilli.

Petrie and O'Brien (1910) fed guinea-pigs with *B. suipestifer* cultures. One died. The rest remained apparently healthy during the period of observation, extending over sixty days, and the bacillus used for feeding was isolated from the excreta on a number of occasions. In this way they produced healthy carriers.

O'Brien (1910) has described an epizootic due to *B. suipestifer* amongst 500 laboratory stock guinea-pigs. All but twenty-one of them died. Five of the survivors proved to be carriers, excreting the bacilli intermittently five months later. The bacilli were, however, of diminished pathogenicity, while spread of infection from these carrier animals did not take place in the few experiments carried out.

It does not appear to be settled how long these bacilli can retain their virulence when unassociated with a definite pathological condition. From analogy with typhoid carriers, it may be for very long periods. On the other hand, outside the animal body Gaertner group bacilli rather readily lose their heat-resisting properties and to some extent their virulence.

It is probable that the virulence of the infecting bacillus, as well as the number present, is important in initiating infection. Meat poisoning outbreaks are far more prevalent in the summer months. This is no doubt in part a question of dosage, since the rate of multiplication of these bacilli is greatly favoured by a high temperature. It is, however, possible that in hot weather the virulence of Gaertner bacilli is raised and carrier bacilli, usually of too low virulence to infect, may become definitely pathogenic to man. It must be remembered that while true Gaertner group bacilli are very virulent by subcutaneous or intraperitoneal injection, they are far less virulent by the mouth, the way that human infection in food poisoning outbreaks is transmitted.

A point which merits careful attention, but which cannot be said to be settled, is the extent to which rats and mice may serve as vehicles for the spread of Gaertner group bacilli and as a source of specific contamination of food. In Addenda II and III, Chapter VI, it has been pointed out that these animals are infected not infrequently with bacilli of this group, while certain members of the group (Danysz bacillus, Rattin, *B. typhi murium*, etc.) are extensively employed to destroy rats and mice. Two possible sources of human infection have therefore to be considered, i.e. direct infection of man through the use of these viruses and specific contamination of the food from the access to it of rats or mice which are infected with Gaertner group bacilli.

The Gaertner bacilli used for the destruction of rats and mice are evidently of low virulence to man, since very few accidents appear to have occurred when compared with the very extensive facilities offered for infection during handling and in use.

Many observers, e.g. Bonhoff (1904), Danysz (1909), etc., advance the view that these organisms are not a danger to man.

Several groups of cases abroad and one outbreak in this country have been ascribed to their use. The English outbreak occurred in the City of London and may be briefly described.

In July, 1908 (Collingridge, 1908), an outbreak of illness occurred at a large business establishment where a considerable number of persons of both sexes were employed. Between the 18th and 22nd twelve men became seriously ill, the symptoms being fever, severe headache, vomiting, diarrhoea, cramp in the abdomen, giddiness, with severe collapse in many cases. There were no deaths. The severe symptoms lasted about forty-eight hours but each case recovered and practically was convalescent at the end of the week.

All those taken ill had their meals in the same dining room and no illness arose amongst those using the other four dining rooms. No article of food was served exclusively in this particular dining room. In the course of the investigation an offensive smell was noticed in the dining room used by the patients, and on removing some of the floor boards on July 30th the bodies, more or less decomposed, of forty mice were found. It was then ascertained that on July 16th some "Liverpool Virus" rat poison had been put down in the dining room and in one of the pantries. Only one tube was used and it was only put down once.

Specimens of the stools of some of the patients were bacteriologically examined by Klein who isolated a bacillus (microbe S.) from the stools which agglutinated the sera of five of the cases tested when convalescent. This microbe S. was pathogenic to a guinea-pig and culturally was identical with the Liverpool virus, both organisms in Klein's opinion showing minute cultural differences from *B. enteritidis*.

It is, however, noteworthy that the sera of the convalescent cases showed only very feeble agglutination reactions with the Liverpool virus or with *B. enteritidis*.

Bainbridge (1909) has shown that the Liverpool virus is indistinguishable from *B. enteritidis* by cultural, agglutination and absorption tests, so that the failure of the sera of these convalescent cases to agglutinate either the Liverpool virus or *B. enteritidis* throws grave doubts upon the etiological association.

The cultural tests used by Klein were insufficient to distinguish microbe S. from the para-Gaertner bacilli, and it is not clear whether this organism was a para-Gaertner bacillus or a true Gaertner organism such as *B. suipestifer.*

The outbreak is of great interest but the available evidence both on bacteriological and epidemiological grounds is insufficient to prove that it was caused by the rat virus.

Mayer (1905) during an investigation of mouse typhoid was himself taken violently ill. *B. typhi murium* was isolated from his excreta while his blood agglutinated this bacillus in high dilution. His acute illness was no doubt due to infection with this organism.

Schibayama (1907) in Japan has described five outbreaks in man all associated with the use of *B. typhi murium* as a virus. Two of them may be mentioned in detail. In one, in April, 1905, thirty persons were attacked with gastro-intestinal symptoms, and three died, twelve to forty-eight hours after eating cooked vegetables. The vegetables were cooked in a wooden vessel which two days earlier had been used to mix the mouse virus (consisting of *B. typhi murium*) with warm water before distribution and which had not subsequently been cleaned out. Seventeen of the cases occurred following eating the freshly cooked vegetables and twelve after eating next day the vegetables left unconsumed. Bacilli isolated from the intestinal contents of the fatal cases, from some of the recovered cases and from the vegetables were found to be completely identical with one another and with *B. typhi murium.*

In another outbreak which occurred in May, 1906, in a Japanese village a peasant brought home the virus mixed with meal. Six children found and ate it in mistake for cake. Next day all were ill with high temperature and diarrhoea. One child of four years died but the others recovered.

Langer and Thomann (1914) describe an outbreak of eleven cases of food poisoning with two deaths due to eating a meat pasty. What they describe as *B. paratyphosus B* was isolated from the internal organs of the cases, and this bacillus was agglutinated by paratyphoid serum and by the serum of the cases. From the flour used they isolated

B. paratyphosus B. The different meal dealers were investigated and the only possible source of infection which could be found was from one of them who also stored a mouse-typhoid preparation. The bait used was identical with *B. paratyphosus B.* The last mouse destruction experiment had been about four months before the beginning of the outbreak, but the authors showed experimentally that the bacilli lived easily for four months in the meal.

It is of interest to note that this virus has set up disease in animals. Thus Krickendt (1901) reported that upon a certain estate the remainder of the mouse-typhoid cultures used against mice became mixed with the food given to calves. A number of calves (four to seven months old) fell ill with symptoms of gastro-enteritis found to be due to *B. typhi murium.* The older animals recovered but the younger died.

Hübener quotes Pfeiffers as finding fever, diarrhoea and loss of appetite to follow the feeding of three sheep with this bacillus. Two died while the third was severely ill.

It is evident that much fuller information is desirable in regard to the use of these rat and mice viruses, and particularly as to how far those handling them develop slight infections with the presence of agglutinins in the blood.

In view of the fact explained in Chapter VI that rats may recover from infection with Gaertner group bacilli and may harbour the bacilli subsequently for long periods, in conjunction with the extensive way in which these rodents infect food, it seems a highly probable hypothesis that the vehicle of infection in some cases is likely to have been rats or mice. From the nature of things it is not possible to supply direct proof of such transmission in any particular outbreak.

Actual mode of infection of the food.

It has yet to be considered how the food becomes infected with Gaertner group bacilli. When the vehicle of infection is meat derived from an animal suffering from disease caused by a Gaertner group bacillus, then of course there is no difficulty, but in considerably more than half the outbreaks this is not the case. For these outbreaks to complete the inquiry we need to explain how the food, frequently not meat at all, became specifically infected, for example, the path whereby the bacilli become transmitted from the animal intestine to the incriminated food.

The study of recorded outbreaks as a rule reveals no data on this point, but for most of them there is definite evidence of the existence of insanitary conditions facilitating infection. In many cases, for example, the food was put to cool after cooking in places exposed to faecal contamination. Such exposure takes many different forms. In some the instruments used to cut up the slaughtered animals were the same as those used for the prepared foods, in others the persons who handled and dressed the carcases, and in some cases also indulged in gut scraping, were employed to prepare and handle the food used for human consumption. In other instances there was much exposure to dust, while for nearly all there was liability to infection from flies, some of which may have been specifically infected.

As regards flies Graham-Smith (1914) found that with flies infected with *B. enteritidis* this organism can be found in the contents of their crops and intestines for at least seven days after infection. Such flies for several days readily infected with this bacillus media plates over which they walked, infection probably being due to inoculation from the proboscis of the fly. The only recorded instance of the recovery of Gaertner group bacilli from flies under natural conditions, of which the writer is aware, is that recorded by Nicoll (1911). This investigator isolated *B. paratyphosus B* from two flies, in one case from the external surface and from the intestine and in the second from the intestine alone. Nicoll concluded that the flies must have carried the bacilli for at least eleven and fourteen days respectively.

The bacteria isolated from flies by Horn and Huber (1911) and described by them as of the paratyphoid group cannot be accepted as true *B. paratyphosus B* organisms.

The cumulative evidence incriminating flies as the vehicle of infection in typhoid fever and all enteritis diseases is very strong, and therefore there is a strong presumption for associating them with the causation of food poisoning infections.

The importance of rats and mice as a vehicle of infection has already been insisted upon. Undoubtedly these animals gain access to food very extensively, and their rôle as transmitting agents is possibly underestimated.

With the above well-known methods of infection available which have been generally accepted as operative for typhoid-dysentery infections it is not necessary to postulate any special and peculiar methods for food poisoning outbreaks.

In the list of recorded outbreaks it will be noted that in several instances the vehicle of infection was meat which had been salted. It is therefore of importance to consider the extent to which salt solutions can eliminate Gaertner group bacilli.

In a series of experiments with commercial brines and artificial salt solutions the writer (Savage, 1910) showed that a rapid elimination of both Gaertner and *B. coli* bacilli took place, at all the temperatures tested, in solutions containing 15 per cent. or more of salt. In 10 per cent. salt solutions the death of the bacilli was also rapid, but less so than for more concentrated solutions. In one experiment with 10 per cent. brine, however, the results showed that when the initial number of bacteria was very large the diminution was very rapid as before, but that a quite small number survived and then, having become acclimatised, were able to live as long as thirty-eight days.

Weichel (1910) also found that salt solutions in a strength of 10 per cent. or over were prejudicial to Gaertner group bacilli added to them, killing the bacilli in a short time. An increase only occurred with a strength of 7 per cent. or less. The actual period of survival varied with the temperature and initial number of bacilli added. On the other hand in meat that already had been infected with food poisoning bacilli before pickling, the killing of the bacilli even with salt solutions up to 19 per cent. takes place after so long a period that pickling as a method for the utilisation of infected meat cannot be considered practicable and this quite apart from the question of toxin production. In meat already infected before pickling the food poisoning bacilli resist killing in 12 to 19 per cent. salt up to seventy-five days, while in a solution of 10 to 13 per cent. numerous food poisoning bacteria within the meat were alive up to eighty days.

Karaffa-Korbutt (1912) studied the inhibitory rather than the killing property of salt solutions. He showed that solutions of 6 to 7 per cent. inhibited the growth of *B. enteritidis*, *B. paratyphosus B*, and *B. aertrycke*.

BIBLIOGRAPHY FOR CHAPTERS V, VI AND X.

The literature of the Gaertner group is very extensive. The undermentioned list only includes those consulted which are referred to in the text and which illustrate special points.

Abraham (1906). *Münch. med. Wochenschrift.* LIII. 2466.
Acomb (1915). *Special Report to Newport (Mon.) Borough Council* (Outbreak No. 102).
Andreijew (1910). *Arb. aus d. Kais. Gesund.* XXXIII. 363.
Angus (1916). *Journ. Roy. Sanitary Inst.* XXXVII. 6. (Outbreak No. 103.)
Aumann (1911). *Centralb. f. Bakt.* I Abt. Orig. LVII. 310.
Bahr, Raebiger and Grosso (1909). *Zeit. f. Infekt. der Haustiere,* v. 295.
Bainbridge (1909). *Journ. of Path. and Bact.* XIII. 443.
—— (1911). *Proc. Roy. Soc. of Med.* IV. (Epidem. Section), 51.
—— (1912). *Lancet,* 1912, March 16, 23, 30.
—— and O'Brien (1911). *Journ. of Hygiene,* XI. 68.
—— and Dudfield (1911). *Ibid.* XI. 24.
Ballard (1890). *Report of Medical Officer L.G.B.* 1890, 189.
Barker (1899). *Brit. Med. Journ.* II. 1367. (Outbreak No. 26.)
Basenau (1894). *Archiv f. Hyg.* XXXII. 219.
Batten and Forbes (1908). *Proc. Roy. Soc. of Med.* I. (Clinical Sec.), 81.
Baumgarten's Jahresbericht (1896), XII. 496 (contains a good account of several Psittacosis outbreaks).
Bernhardt (1913). *Zeit. f. Hyg.* LXXIII. 65.
Bernstein and Fish (1916). *Journ. Am. Med. Assoc.* LXVI. 167.
Berry (1907). *Special Report,* February, 1907. (Outbreak No. 40.)
Böhme (1906). *Zeit. f. Hyg.* LII. 97.
Bonhoff (1904). *Archiv f. Hyg.* L. 222.
Bowes and Ashton (1898). *Brit. Med. Journ.* II. 1457. (Outbreak No. 22.)
Boycott (1906). *Journ. of Hygiene,* VI. 33.
Bradley (1912). *Journ. and Proc. Roy. Soc. N S. Wales,* XLVI. 74.

Brown, J. P. (1915). *Report on outbreak of Food Poisoning at Bacup, June*, 1915.
Brown, G. A. (1906). *Annual Report of M. O. H. Partick*. (Outbreak No. 37.)
—— (1907). *Ibid*. (Outbreak No. 42.)
Buchan (1907). *Lancet*, December 7th, 1907. (Outbreak No. 45.)
—— (1910). *Annual Report of Medical Officer of Health, St Helens*. (Outbreak No. 65.)
Buchanan (1896). *Report of Medical Officer L.G.B.* 1896–7, 115.
Carey (1916). *Am. Journ. Public Health*, VI. 124 (Feb.).
Cathcart (1906). *Journ. of Hyg.* VI. 112.
Christiansen (1917). *Centralb f. Bakt.* 1 Abt. Orig. LXXIX. 196.
Ciurea (1912). *Zeit. f. Infekt. Krank. und Hyg. d. Haust.* XII. 321.
Collingridge (1908). *Report M.O.H. City of London*, 1908.
Dammann and Stedefeder (1910). *Arch. f. Tierheilkunde*, XXXVI. 432.
Danysz (1900). *Annales de l'Inst. Pasteur*, XIV. 193.
—— (1904). *Brit. Med. Journ.* I. 947.
—— (1909). *Ibid.* I. 1909.
Davies, Heaven and Walker Hall (1917). *Public Health*, XXX. 226.
Dean (1911). *Journ. of Hyg.* XI. 259.
Delépine (1903). *Ibid.* III. 68. (Outbreak No. 16.)
Dorset, Bolton and McBryde (1904). *21st Annual Report of the Bureau of Animal Industry*, 138.
Durham (1898). *Brit. Med. Journ.* II. 600. (Outbreak No. 20.)
—— (1898). *Ibid.* II. 1797.
—— (1899). *Trans. of the Path. Soc. of London*, L. 262.
Eberson (1915). *Journ. of Inf. Diseases*, XVII. 331.
Ecker (1917). *Ibid.* XXI. 541.
Fischer (1902). *Zeit. f. Hyg.* XXXIX. 447.
—— (1915). *Centralb. f. Bakt.* Orig. LXXVII. 6.
Ford (1905). *Medical News*, LXXXVI. 1126.
Gaffky (1892). *Deutsch. med. Woch.* XVIII. 297.
Gärtner (1888). *Breslauer ärztl. Ztg.* X. 249.
Gildemeister and Baerthlein (1915). *Arb. a. d. Kais. Gesund.* XLVIII. 122.
Good and Corbett (1913). *Journ. of Inf. Dis.* XIII. 53.
Grabert (1907). *Zeit. f. Infekt. der Haustiere*, III. 218.
Graham-Smith (1914). *Flies in relation to Disease (Non blood-sucking Flies)*. Cambridge University Press.
Hamilton (1912). *Annual Report M.O.H. Eccles*. (Outbreak No. 85.)
Handson and Williams (1908). *Brit. Med. Journ.* II. 1547.
Hay (1910). *Public Health*, XXIII. 181. (Outbreak No. 56.)
Heaven (1909). *Annual Report M.O.H. Bristol*. (Outbreak No. 61.)
Henry (1900). *Annual Report M.O.H. Rochdale*. (Outbreak No. 27.)
Heuser (1910). *Zeit. f. Hyg.* LXV. 8.
Horn and Huber (1911). *Zeit. f. Infekt. der Haust.* X. 443.

Horn and Huber (1912). *Centralb. f. Bakt.* Orig. LXI. 452.
Howarth and Delépine (1902). *Special Report on Derby food poisoning outbreak.* (Outbreak No. 32.)
Hübener (1908). *Deutsch. med. Woch.* XXXIV. 1044.
—— (1910). *Fleischvergiftungen und Paratyphus-infektionen,* Jena, 1910.
Hutchens and Tulloch (1914). *Journ. of Path. and Bact.* XVIII. 431.
Jensen (1913). Kolle und Wassermann, *Handbuch der Pathogenen Microorganismen,* VI. 121. Article, "Kalbërruhr."
Jex-Blake and Wilson (1918). *Brit. Med. Journ.* II. 310.
Joest (1907). *Bericht über die tierärztliche Hochschule zu Dresden für 1906.* Dresden, 1907, 110.
—— (1914). *Zeitschr. f. Infektionskr. der Haust.* L. 307.
Jordan, E. O. (1917). *Journ. of Inf. Diseases,* XX. 457.
—— (1918 a). *Ibid.* XXII. 252.
—— (1918 b). *Ibid.* XXII. 511.
Jordan and Victorson (1917). *Ibid.* XXI. 554.
Karaffa-Korbutt (1912). *Zeit. f. Hyg.* LXXI. 161.
Kerr and Hutchens (1914). *Proc. Royal Soc. of Med.* VII. (Epidem. Section), 171.
Kilborne and Smith (1893). *U.S. Board of Agriculture,* 1893.
Klein (1893). *Journ. of Path. and Bact.* II. 214.
—— (1905). *Trans. Path. Society,* LVI. 132.
Kosche (1906). *Arb. a. d. Kais. Gesund.* XXIV. 181.
Krickendt (1901). *Archiv f. Tierheilk.* XXVII.
Krumwiede and Kohn (1917). *Journ. of Med. Research,* XXXVI. 509.
—— Kohn and Valentine (1918). *Ibid.* XXXVIII. 89.
—— Pratt and Kohn (1916 a). *Ibid.* XXXIV. 355.
—— —— —— (1916 b). *Ibid.* XXXV. 52.
Kutscher and Meinicke (1906). *Zeit. f. Hyg.* LII. 301.
Langer and Thomann (1914). *Deut. med. Woch.* XL. 493.
Ledschbor (1909). *Zeit. f. Infekt. der Haustiere,* VI. 380.
Lewis (1911). *Med. Officer's Report L.G.B.* 1910–11, 314.
Lignières and Zabala (1905). *Rec. Véterinaire,* LXXXII.
—— (1905). *Bull. Soc. Centr. de Méd. Vét. Paris,* LIX. 453.
MacConkey (1906). *Journ. of Hygiene,* VI. 570. (Outbreak No. 31.)
Manninger (1913). *Centralb. f. Bakt.* 1 Abt. Orig. LXX. 12.
Mayer (1908). *Münch. med. Woch.* LV. 2218.
—— (1905). *Münch. med. Woch.* No. 47.
McClintock, Boxmeyer and Siffer (1905). *Journ. of Inf. Diseases,* II. 351.
McClure (1913). *Public Health,* XXVI. 297. (Outbreak No. 88.)
McWeeney (1909). *Brit. Med. Journ.* May, 1909, 1171.
—— (1911). *Journ. of Meat and Milk Hygiene,* I. 1, 65, 129, 192.
—— (1916). *Brit. Med. Journ.* II. 451.
Meissner and Berge (1917). *Deutsche tierärztl. Woch.*

Meissner, Berge and Kohlstock (1912). *Centralb. f. Bakt.* 1 Abt. Orig. LXV. 38.
Meyer (1916). *Journ. of Inf. Diseases,* XIX. 700.
—— and Boerner (1913). *Journ. of Med. Research,* XXIX. 325.
—— Traum and Roadhouse (1916). *Journ. Am. Vet. Med. Assoc.* XLIX. 17.
M'Gowan (1915). *The Pathology and Epidemiology of Swine Fever.* Report issued by Edinburgh and East of Scotland College of Agriculture.
—— (1917). *A further contribution to the Pathology and Epidemiology of Swine Fever.* Report issued by Edinburgh and East of Scotland College of Agriculture.
Mohler and Buckley (1902). *19th Annual Report of the Bureau of Animal Industry, U.S.A.*
Morgan (1905). *Brit. Med. Journ.* 1. 1257.
—— (1906). *Ibid.* 1. 908.
Mori (1905). *Centralb. f. Bakt.* 1 Abt. Orig. XXXVIII. 42.
Mühlens, Darm and Fürst (1908). *Centralb. f. Bakt.* 1 Abt. Orig. XLVIII. 1.
Müller (1914). *Münch. med. Woch.* LXI. 471.
—— (1918). *Centralb. f. Bakt.* 1 Abt. Orig. LXXXI. 505.
Nankivell (1913). *Public Health,* XXVI. 114. (Outbreak No. 87.)
Nason (1899). *Brit. Med. Journ.* II. 791. (Outbreak No. 24.)
Neukirch (1918). *Zeit. f. Hygiene,* LXXXV. 103.
Newman (1908). *Public Health,* XX. 310. (Outbreak No. 39.)
Nicoll (1911). *Journ. of Hygiene,* XI. 381.
De Nobele (1898). *Ann. Soc. de Méd. de Gand,* LXXVII. 281.
O'Brien (1910). *Journ. of Hygiene,* X. 231.
Packer (1900). *Brit. Med. Journ.* II. 1372. (Outbreak No. 28.)
Pappenheimer and Wedel (1914). *Journ. Inf. Dis.* XIV. 180.
Parkes (1905). *Brit. Med. Journ.* II. 1330.
Peck and Thomson (1911). *Special Report on an Outbreak of Food Poisoning in Chesterfield,* 1911.
Penfold (1911). *Proc. Roy. Soc. of Med.* (Path. Sec.), IV. 97.
Perry and Tidy (1919). *Special Report* (Series No. 24) *to the Medical Research Committee.*
Petrie and O'Brien (1911). *Journ. of Hygiene,* X. 287.
—— (1910). *Proc. Roy. Soc. of Med.* IV. 70.
Pitt (1909). *Centralb. f. Bakt.* 1 Abt. Orig. XLIX. 593.
Pottevin (1905). *Ann. de l'Inst. Pasteur,* XIX. 426.
Prigge and Sachsmüke (1909). *Klin. Jahrb.* XXI. 225.
—— (1909). *Ibid.* XXII. 237.
Rappin (1913). *Compt. rend. de la Soc. de Biologie,* LXXV. 410.
Reinhardt and Seibold (1912 a). *Centralb. f. Bakt.* 1 Abt. Orig. LXVI. 59.
—— (1912 b). *Zeit. f. Inf. Krankl. und Hyg. der Haust.* XII. 332.
Reinhold (1912). *Correspondenz-blatt für Schweizer Aerzte,* LXII. 281,332.

Ridder (1909). *Berlin klin. Woch.* XLVI. 2232.

Riemer (1908). *Centralb. f. Bakt.* I Abt. Orig. XLVII. 169.

Rimpau (1908). *Deut. med. Woch.* XXXIV. 1045.

—— (1911). *Arb. a. d. Kais. Gesund.* XXXVIII. 348.

Rolly (1906). *Münch. med. Woch.* LIII. p. 1798.

Rommeler (1909). *Centralb. f. Bakt.* I Abt. Orig. L. 505.

Russ and Trawinski (1918). *Zeit. f. Haust. und Inf.* LXXXV. 32.

Sacquépée (1909). *Les Empoisonnements Alimentaires*, Paris, 1909.

—— and Bellot (1910). *Le progrès médicale*, XXVI. 25.

Savage (1905). *Journ. of Path. and Bact.* X. 341.

—— (1907). *Med. Officer's Report L.G.B.* 1906–7, 253.

—— (1908 a). *Ibid.* 1907–8, 425.

—— (1908 b). *Journ. of Royal San. Instit.* XXIX. 366.

—— (1909). *Med. Officer's Report L.G.B.* 1908–9, 316.

—— (1910). *Ibid.* 1909–10, 446.

—— (1912). *Journ. of Hygiene*, XII. 1.

—— (1913). *Report to the Local Government Board on Bacterial Food Poisoning and Food Infections*, pp. 80. (Food Reports, No. 18.)

—— (1918 a). *Journ. of Hygiene*, XVII. 20.

—— (1918 b). *Ibid.* XVII. 34.

—— and Gunson (1908). *Journ. of Hygiene*, VIII. 601. (Outbreak No. 46.)

—— and Read (1913). *Ibid.* XII. 343.

—— and Forbes (1918). *Ibid.* XVII. 460.

Scarisbrick (1911). *The Medical Officer*, May, 277. (Outbreak No. 76.)

Schellhorn (1910). *Centralb. f. Bakt.* I Abt. Orig. LIV. 428.

Schern (1909). *Arb. a. d. Kais. Gesund.* XXX. 575.

—— (1910). *Ibid.* XXXIII. 387.

—— and Stange (1914). *Zeit. f. Infekt. der Haustiere*, XV. 107.

—— (1914). *Ibid.* XV. 341.

Schibayama (1907). *Münch. med. Woch.* LIV. 979.

Schmidt (1907). *Deutsche tierärztliche Woch.* XVI. 685.

Seiffert (1909). *Zeit. f. Hyg.* LXIII. 273.

Selter (1916). *Ibid.* LXXXI. 387.

Sergeant (1908). *Special Report of Lancashire C.M.O.H.* (Outbreak No. 47.)

—— (1914). *Ibid.* (Outbreak No. 95.)

Smith and Reagh (1903). *Journ. of Med. Research*, IX. 270.

Sobernheim (1910). *Centralb. f. Bakt.* Ref. XLVII. Beit. zu Abteil. 170.

—— and Seligmann (1910). *Zeit. f. Immunitätforschung.* Orig. VI. 401.

Tartakowsky, Nocard et Lechlaenche. *Les maladies microbiennes des animaux.*

Ten Broeck (1916). *Journ. Exp. Med.* XXIV. 213.

—— (1917). *Ibid.* XXVI. 437.

Thomassen (1897). *Ann. de l'Inst. Pasteur*, XI. 523.

Tiberti (1908). *Zeit. f. Hyg.* LX. 41.

—— (1911). *Lo Sperimentale,* 195.

Titze and Weichel (1909). *Deutsche tierärztl. Woch.* 1909.

—— (1909–10). *Arb. a. d. Kais. Gesund.* XXXIII. 516.

Torrey and Rahl (1912). *Journ. of Med. Research,* XXVII. 291.

Trautmann (1902). *Zeit. f. Hyg.* XLIV.

—— (1903). *Ibid.* XLV. 139.

Trawinski (1917). *Ibid.* LXXXIII. 117.

—— (1918). *Centralb. f. Bakt.* Orig. LXXX. 339.

Trommsdorff, Rajchman and Porter (1911). *Journ. of Hygiene,* XI. 89. (Outbreak No. 69.)

Uhlenhuth (1909). *Centralb. f. Bakt.* Ref. XLIV. Beiheft.

—— (1911). *Journ. Roy. Inst. of Public Health,* XIX. 577.

—— and Haendel (1913). Article "Schweinepest und Schweineseuche," Kolle und Wassermann's *Handbuch,* II. Part VI.

—— and Hübener (1908). *Medizinische Klinik,* November 29th, 1823.

—— —— (1908). *Arb. a. d. Kais. Gesund.*

—— Hübener, Xylander and Bohtz (1908). *Arb. a. d. Kais. Gesund.* XXVII. 425.

Ulrich (1906). *Zeit. f. Hyg.* LIII. 176.

United States Dep. of Agric. (1893). *Bureau of Animal Industry Bull.* No. 3, pages 49 and 53.

Van Ermengem (1903). Kolle und Wassermann, *Handbuch der Pathogenen Microorganismen,* II. 637.

Van Heelsbergen (1914). *Centralb. f. Bakt.* I Abt. Orig. LXXII. 38.

—— (1914). *Zeitschr. f. Infekt. der Haustiere,* XVI. 195.

Weichel (1910). *Arb. a. d. Kais. Gesund.* XXXIV. 247.

Weiss (1916). *Proc. of the New York Pathol. Soc.* XVI. 139.

Williams (1910). *Journ. Roy. Instit. of Public Health,* XVIII. 725. (Outbreak No. 69.)

Williams, Murray and Rundle (1910). *Lancet,* II. 730.

Willoughby (1906). *Public Health,* XVIII. 626. (Outbreak No. 35.)

Winzer (1911). *Zeit. f. Fleisch- und Milch-hyg.* XXII. 81. (Abstract in *Journ. of Comp. Path. and Therap.* XXV. 57.)

Xylander (1908 a). *Arb. a. d. Kais. Gesund.* XXVIII. 145.

—— (1908 b). *Zeit. f. Fleisch- u. Milch-hyg.* May, 241. (Abstract in *Journ. Comp. Path. and Therap.* 1908, XXI. 259.)

Zeller (1909). *Zeit. f. Infekt. der Haustiere,* V. 361.

Zingle (1914). *Ibid.* XV. 268.

Zschiesche (1918). *Centralb. f. Bakt.* I Abt. Orig. LXXX. 351.

Zweifel (1911). *Ibid.* I. Abt. Orig. LVIII. 115.

Zwick (1909). *Ibid.* XLIV. Ref. Beiheft. 132.

—— and Weichel (1910). *Arb. a. d. Kais. Gesund.* XXXIII. 250.

—— —— (1910). *Ibid.* XXXIV. 391.

—— —— (1911). *Ibid.* XXXVIII. 327.

CHAPTER XI

Part I. Introduced mainly in connection with processes of manufacture.

FOODSTUFFS being so varied in nature and frequently so diverse in origin and methods of preparation, it is obvious that there is a considerable possibility that in one way or another an extensive range of harmful chemical substances may be introduced. In practice, however, not a large number have been detected, the most important being salts of arsenic, tin, lead, and occasionally barium.

Arsenic. Arsenical compounds are widely diffused in nature, and although minute traces are not uncommon in many foods, or in materials either used as food or for the preparation of food, it was not until the extensive and widespread outbreak of arsenical poisoning in 1900 directed special attention to the subject that the danger of arsenic in food was realized and in any degree adequately investigated. This outbreak so well illustrates the dangers of chemical food contamination from sources not immediately concerned with food production and has been so fully investigated by a Royal Commission (1901) that it is instructive and important to consider it in some detail.

During the latter part of 1900 there occurred in England and Wales exceptional sickness and deaths attributable to poisoning by arsenic. This sickness, which assumed epidemic proportions, principally affected districts in Lancashire and Staffordshire but was not confined to those counties. The total number of persons attacked was at least 6000 and probably the number was very considerably higher.

The evidence showed conclusively that the epidemic was attributable to beer which had become contaminated with arsenic at numerous breweries. In every case the beer was supplied from particular breweries and all of them used brewing sugars (i.e. glucose and invert sugar) supplied by a single firm. These two sugars are extensively used in breweries as adjuncts to, or as partial substitutes for, malt and as priming solutions which are added after the fermentation of the wort. The quantities of arsenic detected in specimens of these sugars was relatively large, and were found by different chemists to vary from 0·008 to 0·131 per cent. (0·56 to 9·17 grains per lb.) in the glucose and from 0·02 to 0·062 per cent. (1·4 to 4·34 grains per lb.) in the invert sugar, all estimated as arsenious oxide.

This heavy contamination with arsenic was traced to the use, by the firm implicated, of sulphuric acid all supplied from one firm of acid makers. The amount of arsenic in this acid was found to be exceptionally high, amounts varying from 1·4 to 2·6 per cent. of arsenious oxide being found by different analysts.

The firm supplying the arsenical sulphuric acid did not inform the firm making the brewing sugars that their acid contained arsenic, and stated in their evidence that they did not know the purpose for which it was required.

The proportions of glucose and invert sugar used in the preparation of the disease-producing beers were as a general rule no greater than those which are used in many other English breweries. The amounts of arsenic present in the beers brewed with the contaminated sugars must have varied greatly at different breweries and in different kinds of beers since the proportions of these sugars used varied considerably, while material differences would result due to the stage at which the sugar was introduced into the beer. As a rule the proportion of arsenic in the beers actually used was probably 0·25 to 1 grain per gallon or even less, although in exceptional cases amounts as high as 1·5 and 3 grains per gallon were detected.

While some of the sufferers were moderate beer drinkers the majority seem to have been heavy drinkers of this beverage.

As was to be anticipated, in view of the great variations in dosage and the duration of the period over which arsenical beer was drunk and the differences between individual beer drinkers as regards age, sex, conditions of nutrition and habits as regards alcohol, the disease produced by the arsenical beer during the epidemic varied greatly in its manifestations.

There occurred throughout the epidemic, and particularly towards its termination, an abundance of cases with symptoms corresponding to those described as characteristic of sub-acute poisoning by arsenic. "They showed, for example, inflammation of various mucous surfaces leading to coryza, huskiness, lachrymation and the like; gastro-intestinal disturbances and diarrhoea; peripheral neuritis affecting sensory and motor nerves and in some cases associated with herpes or with well-marked erythromelagia; keratosis; or recent pigmentation corresponding to that which not infrequently occurs in persons taking arsenic for long periods." In addition numerous cases were met with in which these kinds of symptoms were slight or absent altogether.

The Royal Commission found it impossible to determine with any accuracy the number of fatal cases, but seventy were definitely recorded from this cause, and undoubtedly this was only part of the total.

The outbreak naturally directed the attention of the Commissioners to other possible ways in which arsenic may gain access to beer, and they reported that small quantities might be derived from malt, the grain being exposed when on the kiln to the products of combustion of fuel containing arsenical materials, and from chemical substances used, other than sugars, containing minute quantities of arsenic.

In nearly every case samples of brewing sugars from other sources were found arsenic-free, and the Commissioners concluded that arsenic-free beer was practicable.

As regards the presence of arsenic in beer before the outbreak, the Royal Commissioners state "There can be no doubt that a considerable proportion of beer brewed in some parts of the country before 1900 contained noteworthy quantities of arsenic, mainly derived from malt and from brewing sugars."

An outbreak of about fourteen cases at Halifax in 1902 was

traced to beer containing arsenic and the evidence pointed strongly to the conclusion that the implicated beers had been contaminated by arsenic derived from malt used in their preparation. In nearly every instance the malt concerned had been dried over local gas coke, and malt dried in this way was found in the 1901 inquiries to be especially liable to contain arsenic.

The Commissioners expressed the opinion that much of the alcoholic neuritis occurring among beer drinkers before 1900, and particularly in localities such as Manchester, was attributable to arsenic in beer.

The Commissioners considered that the exclusion of small quantities of arsenic from food and drink is of greater importance than might at first sight be supposed. Clinically the effect of quite small quantities of arsenic administered over long periods with food cannot be said to have been fully studied: evidence of marked toxicity may be absent, but yet the arsenic may have unrecognized effects upon nutrition. They add "it would be unwise to express an opinion that any quantity of arsenic, however small, is to be regarded as admissible in any article of food, and we think it should be the aim of the food manufacturer to exclude arsenic altogether from his products."

It is well known that in the past arsenical poisoning has been caused by the consumption of sweets coloured with arsenical pigments, but this crude form of poisoning is probably a thing of the past. That arsenic may, however, gain access to sweets from other sources, although probably of very rare occurrence, is shown by the interesting outbreak in Manchester in 1908, carefully described by J. R. Hutchinson (1910).

In this outbreak sixty-two known cases of poisoning occurred, fifty-six in children attending four schools, five in children under school age and one in an adult, the mother of one of the children attacked. Fortunately the amount of arsenic in the sweets was so large that in all cases vomiting was promptly caused and, after a transient illness, all the sufferers were quickly well again, usually the same or next day. The symptoms in every case were those of an acute irritant poison with sudden onset with acute vomiting. As a rule this was the only symptom, although abdominal pain was met with in some children and purging in others.

Delépine examined the sweets and found two kinds, distinguished by their physical appearance, one of which was arsenic free, while the other contained as much as an average of 10 to 11 grains of arsenic per pound of sweets. Some of the larger sweets contained probably not less than $\frac{1}{20}$ grain of arsenic in each.

Although detailed inquiries were made into the origin of the arsenic, the source was never satisfactorily ascertained. Glucose entered largely into the composition of the sweets and the probability is that this was the vehicle of conveyance, but this could not be established. If so the glucose must have been very highly contaminated with arsenic.

There are several other sources from which arsenic may get into foods. For example, Smith (1912) has shown that food may be contaminated with small quantities of arsenic from shellac which is used not infrequently as a coating for some kinds of cheap confectionery. It is used as a varnish for different food containers.

The modern spraying of fruits and vegetables with insecticide solutions is another possible source of arsenic and other metals. Arsenic is an ingredient of many insecticide solutions and may gain access to food from this source with want of care. MacFadden (1913–4), for instance, mentions that during 1914 a consignment of apples from the United States had on their skins a bluish deposit, evidently the remains of an insecticide wash. Analysis showed that copper in small quantities and arsenic in traces were present in this deposit.

This subject has recently been investigated by the New Hampshire (U.S.A.) Agricultural Experiment Station (1917) in regard to the use of lead arsenate solution. This report shows that in the case of apples the maximum amount of the poison that may be expected to occur on the fruit would not exceed 0·5 mgm. per apple. In the case of small fruit the possibility of danger is greater and half a pint of strawberries may carry as much as 8 mg. of oxide of arsenic.

Such a dose while insufficient to cause symptoms in an adult in the ordinary way might affect enfeebled adults or children. In the same way green vegetables, such as cabbages or lettuce, may be infected and carry a relatively large amount of poison. Recently arsenic has been found in a considerable number of samples of baking powder substitute (MacFadden, 1916–7). In these samples the ingredients of the baking powder mixture were cream of tartar substitute (acid calcium phosphate, sodium bicarbonate and ground rice). All the arsenic was contained in the acid calcium phosphate. Extensive inquiries were made and arsenic was found in many samples from many different parts of the country. While in the majority of cases the amounts reported were relatively small and, as judged by the limit laid down by the Royal Commission on Arsenical Poisoning (0·01 grain of arsenic per pound, equal to 1·43 parts per million), not calling for special action, in about fifty cases the amounts found reached as much as 400 parts of arsenic per million. One sample of unmixed acid calcium phosphate contained as much as 4·5 grains of arsenic per pound (or 643 parts per million). When traced to the source the poison was found to be derived from sulphuric acid contaminated with arsenic which was used to prepare the acid calcium phosphate.

Antimony. Like arsenic, antimony is widely distributed in nature and is a powerful poison, but the writer is unaware of any outbreaks of poisoning, acute or chronic, from this metal or its salts in food. Pond (1905) showed that the red rubber rings used for mineral water bottles contained large quantities of antimony and that particles of these rings may be ingested with the mineral water. He suggested this as a possible cause of appendicitis, but no evidence of poisoning from this source has been actually reported.

Lead. Lead occurs to a considerable extent in articles brought into close association with food. For example, some of the enamels used for glazing earthenware contain lead, tea is wrapped in lead foil, wine bottles are sometimes cleaned by shaking lead shot in them, soda water siphons are fitted with valves containing lead, cider may be heavily contaminated with lead from vessels used in the course of its manufacture, tins for meat preparations may contain and give up lead.

In all these ways lead may gain access to food and be a cause of chronic poisoning, but few definite recorded cases from these sources have been recorded, except from contaminated cider.

An interesting case was observed by Halenke and reported by him to Lehmann (1902). Two women ate cranberry tart for which they had cooked the cranberries in a cheap earthenware pot. Soon after eating part of the tart they became ill, one severely so. The glaze had been dissolved from the inside of the pot. A piece of the tart contained 160 mg. of lead. It was estimated that each woman had consumed from 400 to 600 mg. of malate of lead and that approximately as much as 1000 mg. had been dissolved in this single cooking.

Cider, which contains malic acid, was at one time responsible for a number of cases of lead poisoning from being allowed to come into contact with lead vats during the process of manufacture. Cases of lead poisoning from this cause were reported as long ago as 1767 by Baker.

Copper. This metal may occur in foods in minute quantities, but very rarely is present in amounts capable of setting up disease symptoms when derived from accidental sources.

In the Report of the Sanitary Department of the German Army for 1894 to 1896 it is recorded (see *British Medical Journal*, 1898, November 12th, p. 1532) that seventy-five men of an infantry regiment were seized with very severe diarrhoea. It was found that all the men attacked had eaten food cooked in copper utensils, and copper was found by chemical analysis both in the fragments left and in the dejecta. The symptoms were those of copper poisoning with the peculiarity that in some cases there was a considerable rise of temperature.

Its intentional addition to foods is dealt with in Chapter XII.

The occasional presence of copper salts in oysters is well known although the popular impression is incorrect that all "green oysters" are so coloured because of the presence of this metal. Bulstrode (1894–5) reported that green oysters from certain Cornish beds contained copper which imparted to them a distinct metallic taste, and Thorpe found that the average amount of copper in these oysters, estimated as cupric oxide, was about 0·02 grains per oyster, the amount, however, showing considerable variation in individual molusks. The metallic taste would discourage consumption, while a considerable number of such oysters would have to be consumed to yield a poisonous dose of copper.

More recently MacFadden (1913–14) reported the presence of considerable amounts of copper and zinc in certain oysters obtained in Liverpool. The analytical results showed that zinc was present on an average in an amount more than double that of the copper found, and MacFadden remarks "if this ratio should prove to be of common occurrence in oysters contaminated by metals of this group it is by no means certain that the protection afforded by abnormal colour and taste would suffice to safeguard consumers against serious risk of metallic poisoning from zinc, the presence of which would not be so obvious."

Part II. Chemicals added from the action of the food upon the retainers in which it is put upon the market.

A striking feature of modern civilization is the extent to which food of various kinds is preserved and sold, not in the fresh condition, but stored in receptacles under conditions which preserve the food in an eatable condition. The amount of food canned is now enormous. For example, Report No. 54, "Canned Foods," of the Department of Commerce, states that in 1914 the value of foods canned in the United States alone amounted to about 258 million dollars, over 103 million cases being packed.

The kinds of foodstuffs canned are very varied, but are mainly condensed milk, meat foods, fish, shellfish, fruits and vegetables.

Nature of the retainers. Writing in 1908 Dr MacFadden (1908) remarks, "Until recent years most of the preserved foods manufactured in this country were packed in tin-plate receptacles. Tin-plate is a convenient material for this purpose, as an efficient seal can easily be procured in vessels made from it and no special disadvantage arises from subjecting them to high temperatures, thus enabling sterilization of their contents to be readily effected. Besides this, tin-packed goods are much more easily and safely transportable, and occupy less storage space than vessels of an equal capacity made from glass or earthenware. For these reasons tin-plate is still used in the packing of almost all preserved foods imported into this country, and also of many of those exported from it. It has been supplanted of late years to a very large extent, however, by glass and earthenware, more especially the former, in the case of goods intended for the home market.

"So much have glass-packed food materials advanced in public favour, that it appears to be profitable for certain home manufacturers to transfer imported canned meats, such as tongues, sardines, etc., from their tin receptacles into glass containers. The fact that a considerable quantity of the preserved food in this country is sold in glass retainers does not therefore exclude the possibility of the food being contaminated with tin, transferred from a tin-plate receptacle."

Metals which gain access. Although iron and lead may gain access in small quantities, the comparative harmlessness of the one and the minute quantities added of the other render contamination with these metals of no practical importance and the only metallic addition of any real significance is tin. The comprehensive report by Buchanan and Schryver (1908) to the Local Government Board gives much information upon this subject and has been largely relied upon for the following facts.

The amount of tin which may be present. The amount found is influenced by the following four factors.

(a) *The nature of the food canned.* Buchanan summing up the matter states "Practically all foods canned in the ordinary way become to some extent contaminated with tin as a result of the contact of the food with the tin-plate of the can. Tin is taken up by meat extracts and essences to a greater extent than by most other meats. This results from the acidity naturally possessed by the meat extractives in these preparations. Certain canned fruits and vegetables, and foods, such as canned soups of which the latter form part, are also specially liable to take up tin from the can in consequence of their natural acidity. Canned peaches, cherries, pears, apricots, pineapples, tomatoes, asparagus, canned fruit puddings, and tomato soup are included in this category. Notable quantities of tin have been found in certain samples of canned lobster.

"In such cases tin may penetrate into the substance of solid foods, and in the case of canned foods which consist of both liquid and solid portions, e.g., canned fruit, the solid portion may come to contain relatively larger proportions of tin than the liquid. This results from the fact that the tin, after solution in the liquid contents of the can, becomes in course of time adsorbed to, or chemically combined with, the solid contents."

This point is of importance since it is usually assumed that the tin is in solution. If separate estimates of the tin in the drained solids and in the liquor be made it will be found that a large proportion of the tin is in an insoluble form. The longer the food has been canned the higher is the proportion of insoluble tin, the tin in solution being slowly rendered insoluble.

Wirthle, for example, found that with preserved meats canned for some time the meat contained three times as much tin as the juice.

As regards the actual amounts found Schryver summarises the results of some 130 analyses of different canned goods, most of which had been kept a considerable time, in the following table:

Foodstuffs containing			Number	Percentage of total
Less than 1 grain per pound	...	...	72	55·4
Between 1 and 2 grains per pound		...	35	26·9
Between 2 and 3 grains per pound		...	17	13·0
More than 3 grains per pound ...		...	6	4·6

Where maxima or minima only are quoted, one maximum number and one minimum number are included in this total.

The very comprehensive report upon selected and representative varieties of canned foods made by an American Technical Committee (1917) gives a good idea of the amounts found, as shown in the following table:

Nature of the food	Average tin contents—maxima and minima (in milligrms per kilo)	Remarks
Michigan apples ...	68—73	Age varied from 1 to 11 months.
New York apples ...	166—175	Only slight increase with time in
Pennsylvania apples ...	63—79	containers.
String beans	85—181	Regular increase with time in containers (4 to 13½ months).
Cider	73—128	Slight increase with storage.
Clam juice	17—34	Very little variation.
Condensed milk ...	5—22	Very little at any time, with slight
Corn	6—25	increase during storage.
Peas	14—-22	No appreciable difference with storage.
Pumpkin	39—666	Wide variations met with. Varied with the kind. Thus New York pumpkins usually contained less than 100 mgrms, while Illinois pumpkins usually 300 to 600. Marked increase with time of storage.
Tomatoes	47—89	Very uniform on the whole as regards amount of tin and very slight increase with storage.
Salmon	36—52	All examined at one age, i.e. 8½ months.
Tuna fish	10—38	At first only 10–15 mgrm. and only increased to 23–38 after 12 months storage.

(b) *The age of the tins, i.e. the period since canning.* The quantity of tin taken up from the can usually increases with the time since canning but varies, as shown in the above table, with the kind of food. In the case of acid foodstuffs, solution seems to take place at a somewhat greater rate during the first few months after canning than at subsequent periods.

(c) *The quality of the tin-plate.* Buchanan states "The quality of tin-plate used for the canning of foods varies very considerably, and there is no doubt that tin-plate is often employed in which the coating of tin has been reduced to a minumum from considerations of cheapness, with the result that a comparatively small erosion will in parts expose the steel or iron of the plate, and thereby facilitate an electrolytic action likely to accelerate the further solution of the tin."

The American Technical Committee paid special attention to this point, which indeed was the main object of their investigation, but found that none of the difficulties encountered, (including such points as perforation of the cans, discoloration of cans or contents, or amount of tin) in the twenty experimental packs of twelve representative foods in plain cans, were eliminated by heavy tin coatings.

(d) *The solder used and the method of soldering.* As Buchanan remarks, "if solder (containing both tin and lead) is allowed to gain access to the interior of the can a very conspicuous solution of tin may take place. A can only a few months old in which this has happened may show a greater degree of tin contamination of its contents than a properly sealed can which has been kept for many years and used for similar material." Contamination by tin in this way is the more serious on account of the simultaneous risk of serious contamination by lead.

The toxicity of tin. Tin may exert a toxic action in two definite ways. The amount taken into the body with the food may be so considerable that a single dose may set up acute symptoms, or chronic poisoning may be induced by much smaller quantities taken over a long period. Schryver (1908) has collected details of a few recorded cases of acute tin poisoning from foodstuffs. They are very few in number and in all the symptoms were those of acute irritant poisoning with rapid onset. He remarks "So far as may be gathered such irritant poisoning has been produced in adults who have taken at a single meal a quantity of tin equal to two grains, or thereabouts. It will also be noticed that in some of these cases the dose has apparently been taken in a small bulk of food, in circumstances which suggest that the proportion of tin present in the food which caused the mischief was rather of the order found in canned foods which owe their metallic contamination to escape of solder than of the kind which may be present in well-soldered tins that are

merely 'old.' At the same time it must be remembered that
it is only the severe cases that are at all likely to receive
investigation and record, and it is impossible to ignore the
probability that taking at a single sitting food which contained the equivalent of 2 grains of tin (or even an amount
materially less than 2 grains) would result in gastro-intestinal disturbance, whether the tin was concentrated in a
small bulk of food or present in a larger mass.

"On the other hand it may be regarded as established by
general experience that canned foods, such as fruits, which
when consumed within a few months of canning must often
contain quantities of tin, such as $\frac{1}{2}$ grain per pound, do not
in ordinary circumstances occasion gastro-intestinal irritation in the amount usually taken at a single meal."

Buchanan summarising this question accepts the view
that this irritant action may result when tin salts are present
in foods in such quantities as may lead to 1 or 2 grains of
tin being taken at a time. The concentration of the tin in
the food, the condition of the stomach at the time the food
was swallowed, the susceptibility of the individual and other
circumstances would no doubt largely govern the result in
individual cases. It is clear that canned foods which are
capable of causing such symptoms contain much larger
amounts of tin than occur in the canned foods ordinarily
supplied for consumption. Buchanan suggests that when
as much as 2 grains to the pound are found, the food should
be regarded with grave suspicion and as "potentially deleterious to health." He also draws attention to the desira-
bility from an administrative point of view of requiring the
date and place of preparation to be shown on the labels or
to be otherwise available when required.

As regards evidence of chronic poisoning Schryver was
unable to trace any instances in which such chronic poisoning
had followed as a result of the continued ingestion, along
with food, of comparative small doses of tin. He experimented upon himself over a period of three weeks, taking
during the first week approximately 1 grain (64·5 mgrm.)
of tin per day, during the second week 2 grains per day and
3 grains per day for the third week. He made careful analyses

of the faeces and urine and found that when the quantities ingested were 1 to 2 grains per day no evidence of accumulation was forthcoming at the end of a fortnight, but that when the amount taken reached 3 grains per day the excretion of the tin did not keep pace with the intake.

Schryver also considered, and discusses in his report, the results of different observers with animal experiments and concluded from all the different investigations that "they do not indicate much probability of serious risk of chronic poisoning by the absorption of non-irritant compounds of tin as a result of a diet which consists largely of canned foods and is continued over considerable periods of time."

The general results recorded above, and others in the literature, do not suggest that tin plays any part of importance in connection with food poisoning acute or chronic.

REFERENCES.

Buchanan and Schryver (1908). *L.G.B. Reports of Inspector of Foods.* No. 7, "On the presence of tin in certain canned foods."

Bulstrode (1894–5). *L.G.B. Report on oyster culture in relation to disease*, 99–108.

Hutchinson, J. R. (1910). *Journ. Roy. Inst. Public Health*, XVIII. 601.

Lehmann (1902). *Hygienische Rund.* XII. 785.

MacFadden (1908). *L.G.B. Reports of Inspector of Foods.* No. 6, "On preservatives in meat foods packed in cans or glass."

—— (1913–4). *L.G.B. Report on the Work of Inspectors of Foods for the year* 1913–4, 106.

—— (1916–7). *L.G.B. Report on the Work of Inspectors of Foods for the year* 1916–7, 6.

New Hampshire Agric. Exper. Station Bulletin 183, June, 1917, and *Journ. Am. Med. Assoc.* 1917, LXIX. 1083.

Pond (1905). *Lancet*, I. 1610.

Report of an Investigation by a Technical Committee representing The National Canners Association, The American Sheet and Tin Plate Company, and The American Can Company: "Relative value of Different Weights of Tin Coating on Canned Food Containers," 1917.

Royal Commission on Arsenical Poisoning, 1901. Part I. *Report;* Part II. *Final Report.*

Smith (1912). *U.S. Dept. Agric. Bureau of Chemistry, Washington.*

Wirthle. *Chem. Zeitschr.* XXIV. 263.

CHAPTER XII

CHEMICALS DELIBERATELY ADDED TO FOOD—
CHEMICAL PRESERVATIVES

THERE are many problems in the realm of preventive medicine which are still the subject of acute controversy and about which wide differences of opinion are held, both as to the actual facts and as to their interpretation. In spite of the large volume of evidence which has been presented, the considerable body of facts which have been collected and the immense mass of more or less hypothetical considerations which have been advanced, the question of the necessity and safety of chemical preservatives in foods yet remains a controversial matter upon which very different opinions are held.

Owing to the perishable nature of foods and the fact that at certain times some are plentiful while at others difficult to get or unobtainable, man, for many centuries and indeed throughout his historical existence, has resorted to forms of food preservation. In addition he found that preservation in some of its forms materially altered the taste and quality of the food and thus gave him new, and frequently more palatable, types of food. With the growth of tribes into nations and of nations from agricultural to industrial communities this necessity of keeping unimpaired the food of seasons of plenty to times of scarcity has been accentuated, while the advantages of enabling rapidly perishable articles to be transported in a good condition from regions of origin to places of consumption have, with industrial concentration of the population, largely extended the practice.

It has come therefore to be a commonplace that a large part of the food of the community is not eaten in its original condition but after various manipulations, all in the direction of preventing bacterial decomposition and so allowing the food to be kept for more or less prolonged periods.

The earlier methods of preservation were largely non-chemical in nature, such as drying or smoking, but the latter is really a chemical process, chemicals, such as creosote, being developed and acting as preservatives. Further developments have been along the lines of using such well-known substances as common salt, sugar and vinegar. The use of nitre (potassium nitrate) may be considered as an example of the employment of a substance intermediate between these older substances and the more modern chemical preservatives.

To these older processes, sanctioned by custom and used without demonstrable harm, no objection on the score of injury to health has been raised, nor can any objection be advanced on this ground to the use of the non-chemical methods of preservation by heat and refrigeration. The controversy has raged round the addition of certain more recently discovered chemical substances specially used as preservatives to prevent bacterial decomposition, and these only need to be discussed here.

Concurrently with this development, chemical substances have come to be also used not to preserve the food, but to enhance its attractiveness, by giving a fictitious appearance of quality, or to pander to a popular prejudice in favour of supplying a food of a particular appearance or colour. This group includes the different colouring matters added to food and such special matters as the addition of copper salts to peas or other vegetables.

The whole subject of preservatives in food cannot be treated here with the detailed consideration which its importance demands, but it will be possible to discuss in the space available the salient considerations and their relationship to food poisoning and food infections. Two extreme attitudes have been adopted amongst others. One party has taken the line that as these chemical preservatives are in the main substances with definite physiological actions upon the human body, causing poisonous symptoms when administered in sufficient doses, therefore they should be entirely excluded from food unless those who wish to add them can adduce evidence sufficient to prove that they are harmless to man. The other extreme view adopts in practice the standpoint that it is for those who object to their introduction to demonstrate their harmfulness and that until this has been done they should be allowed to employ them.

The most obvious fact in the whole controversy is its extreme complicatedness since it involves questions of dosage, the varying reactions of individuals to drugs, problems of elimination under different conditions and the study of a whole series of chemicals, some of which are used in combination, while additions to the list are constantly being made.

Evidence of the prejudicial effect of the addition of these chemical preservatives has been adduced along a number of lines, the following being the most important:

(1)   That the preservative added is itself harmful to man in the amounts found or which may be present.

(2)   That the addition of these preservatives allows the food to be collected, prepared or stored under conditions which are prejudicial to health, such methods being commercially practicable only because the addition of preservatives prevents the food decomposition which these unhygienic practices would render inevitable.

(3)   That while these preservatives in the amounts found may not be harmful to normal man they are likely to be detrimental to certain sections of the community, i.e. the delicate, diseased or young. The cogency of this argument is augmented by the fact that for most foods the law does not require disclosure of the presence or amount of preservatives and that it is therefore impossible to ensure or safeguard in any satisfactory way that such sensitive persons may not be dosed with these chemicals without their consent or knowledge.

(4)   That the fact that our present knowledge may not be sufficient to allow the formulation of conclusive evidence as to harmfulness to be forthcoming does not invalidate the possibility that their administration, especially over prolonged periods, may be a cause of ill health. In other words it is a fair line of argument to take that the addition to food of substances which are known poisons in large doses may

exert a definite, if unknown, effect upon the tissues of the animal organism and so be a cause of chronic disease, and that the public should not be exposed to these unknown, although problematical, risks without their knowledge and consent.

Suggested selective bacterial action of preservatives. In connection with (2) above it has been suggested that chemical preservatives may be peculiarly prejudicial by exerting a selective action on bacteria, restraining the putrefactive and other types which would make the food obtrusively unsound while allowing the more pathogenic bacteria to develop, if not unchecked at least not restrained, to the same extent.

Grünbaum[1], for example, concluded that "The addition of a small quantity of a preservative like borax does not hinder the growth of microorganisms as a whole, although it does repress the putrefactive ones." Bernstein[2] developed this idea, experimenting only with boric acid. He found that this chemical to the extent of 0·3 per cent. (20 grains per pound) prevented objective decomposition while if putrefaction had commenced it inhibited further changes. He found that its inhibitory action was greater against *proteus* organisms than against *B. coli*, and was more marked than its action on *B. typhosus* or *B. enteritidis*. Klein[3] carried out a few experiments in this direction but with a different result, finding that a marked inhibitory action was exhibited by 0·5 per cent. boric acid on both *B. coli* and *B. enteritidis*, but rather less on the latter, in both broth and sausage meat.

The experimental evidence is scanty and very incomplete and does not satisfactorily establish the point, while no experiments appear to have been carried out to test the action of these chemical preservatives upon the putrefactive anaerobes. On general grounds it is unlikely that less resistant organisms, like *B. typhosus* and members of the Gaertner group, should survive in the presence of preservatives better than the hardier saprophytic forms.

Chief preservatives used. The preservatives most commonly

[1] *Brit. Med. Jour.* 1900, II. August 18th.
[2] *Brit. Med. Jour.* 1910, I. April 10th, p. 928.
[3] *Public Health*, 1910, XXIII. p. 438.

employed, in addition to such long-established substances as common salt, sugar, vinegar and nitre, are boric acid and its compounds, salicylic acid and salicylates, sulphurous acid and sulphites, formaldehyde, benzoic acid and benzoates, fluorides and hydrogen peroxide. A number of others have been introduced from time to time but are rarely used. Not infrequently two or more preservatives are used together. These preservatives are frequently sold under fancy names, either as single substances or as mixtures of two or more of them.

Evidence of harmfulness. For details of individual cases of poisoning and the experimental evidence connecting these preservatives with ill health or actual poisoning the reader is referred to the Report of the Departmental Committee on Preservatives and Colouring Matters (1909), Thresh and Porter's book, *Preservatives in Food*, 1906, and the individual papers, as the whole of the evidence cannot be summarised in the space available and any selection of evidence would lead to partial and possibly biased presentation. It is only proposed to discuss the broad general principles.

Most of these substances are admittedly poisonous when administered in large doses and therefore the controversy over their harmfulness ranges over the question of their administration in small doses. For example, for boric acid and its compounds, there are a good many definite recorded cases of poisoning from their use in large amounts. While therefore the direct harmfulness of these substances in small or minimal doses may be difficult to establish, objectors to their use are on firm ground when they take the line that the use of these chemicals should be restricted and controlled in order to prevent the different vendors or manufacturers, through whose hands the food passes, from separately and severally dosing these foodstuffs, with the possibility that the food as consumed may contain a poisonous dose.

Since it is admitted that small quantities only are necessary for food preservation purposes while large quantities are undoubtedly harmful, the position of those who demand that some limits as to amounts present should be imposed is really unassailable. Those who handle these preservatives

are for the most part ignorant of their possibly harmful
character, they are not trained to appreciate the significance
and niceties of small chemical additions and the need for
accuracy, so that in practice it is common to find chemical
preservatives present far in excess of any quantity necessary
to prevent bacterial decomposition[1].

The common practice of selling these food preservatives
under fancy names is a direct inducement to irregularity and
excess of dosage, for those using them frequently have no
idea what substances they are using or their strength, and
rely blindly upon the directions given on the labels.

A further fact of general applicability is that most of
these substances are foreign to the animal body and are
excreted as foreign substances by the kidneys. This organ
is particularly sensitive to chemical substances so secreted,
and it is therefore a reasonable supposition that their elimination may be locally harmful, particularly to those with
defective or damaged kidneys. It is this point which has
induced some authorities to favour the use only of benzoic
acid and benzoates as preservatives since they combine with
glycocol and are excreted in the form of hippuric acid, a
normal and harmless constituent of the urine. As Rosenau[2]
puts it, "we know that the human organism is prepared to take
care and render harmless a certain amount of benzoic acid,
we know that this mechanism is a very efficient one and is
capable of taking care of relatively large amounts of benzoic
acid."

On the other hand the special German Commission in
1913 found that the administration of benzoic acid in repeated and relatively large doses caused in dogs poisonous
symptoms, and, if continued, death. To get this result,
however, as much as 0·4 grm. per pound of body weight had
to be administered.

---

[1] For example, in a sample of brawn the writer found as much as 96
grains per pound of boric acid, and when the brawn-maker was invited to
explain why he used a quantity so vastly in excess of the need he stated
that he thought it was rather hot weather so took a small handful and
mixed it in with the batch. He evidently thought it could be used like
common salt.

[2] *Preventive Medicine and Hygiene*, 1913.

The Departmental Committee on Preservatives and
Colouring Matters (1909) did not arrive at definite opinions
in regard to the harmfulness of most of the preservatives
they considered, as the evidence laid before them was in
some respects conflicting, in many cases partial and incomplete, while no evidence was forthcoming as regards certain
points. The Committee by no means condemned the total use
of all preservatives but recommended restriction in their use.

The views of this Committee largely influence the practice
in this country, so it is important to state some of them and
the following may be quoted as examples:

Sulphites. "Concerning the physiological effects of the
sulphites, a preservative often used by butchers, poultry
dealers and brewers, there has been no evidence laid before
this Committee. It appears, however, that when sulphurous
acid or its salts are added to organic compounds, such as
beer or butcher's meat, some of it is at once oxidized to
sulphate, which may be regarded at any rate in the amount
present as indifferent; some attaches itself chemically to
certain constituents of the food in question and the compound
formed is also innocuous; a third portion remains as sulphurous acid, and it is this portion alone which is of permanent
efficacy as an antiseptic. Concerning the effect of this
moiety upon the consumer pharmacologists do not seem
agreed, and further investigation is required before the
sulphites can be regarded as either harmful or harmless."

As regards this preservative it may however be remarked
that in 1898 the Imperial German Board of Health forbade
the use of sodium sulphite in food on account of its harmfulness, while its use is also prohibited in America by the
Federal Pure Food Act of 1906.

Boron preservatives. "After very carefully weighing the
evidence we have come to the conclusion that as regards
the trade in fresh and cured meat, fish, butter, margarine
and other food substances, in the consumption of which but
small quantities of the antiseptic are taken into the system,
there exists no sufficient reason for interfering to prevent
the use of boron preservatives." As regards milk they
definitely pronounced against their use.

Copper sulphate. This substance is chiefly used in the greening of vegetables. The Departmental Committee remarks "It is highly undesirable that what is admittedly a poisonous substance should be used, even to the smallest extent, in connection with such food as may be consumed in considerable quantity. Direct proof that vegetables containing copper are injurious to the consumer is from the very nature of the case difficult to obtain, and we must admit that we have not succeeded in obtaining it. There is evidence pointing to the conclusion that the copper, when added to the vegetables, forms a compound which is not easily soluble in the human economy. There is, however, evidence of a contrary character, and it is not clear to us that the whole of the copper added becomes, or remains, insoluble under all conditions. Be this as it may, recent events have so incontestably demonstrated the serious and widespread mischief which may result from the consumption of food and drink, other than sweetmeats, containing even minimal quantities of poisonous metallic substances, that we are strongly of opinion that such poisonous substances should be rigorously excluded." As regards the amounts of copper sulphate actually found Dearden[1] gives particulars of twenty-three samples of vegetables analysed at Manchester containing amounts varying from 0·5 to 6 grains of crystallized copper sulphate per pound.

A valuable series of studies upon the influence of vegetables greened with copper salts on the health of man are contained in the Report of the Referee Board of Consulting Scientific Experts appointed by the U.S.A. Department of Agriculture[2].

This report contains a detailed account of the experimental investigations conducted upon both man and animals. The general conclusions of the Referee Board are as follows:

"(a) Copper salts used in the colouring of vegetables as in commercial practice cannot be said to reduce, or lower, or injuriously affect the quality or strength of such vegetables, as far as the food value is concerned."

---

[1] *Public Health*, 1910, XXIII. p. 426.
[2] *U.S. Dept. of Agric.* 1913, Report No. 97.

" (b)　Copper salts used in the greening of vegetables may have the effect of concealing inferiority, inasmuch as the bright green colour imparted to the vegetables simulates a state of freshness they may not have possessed before treatment."

" (c)　In attempting to define a large daily quantity of copper, regard must be had to the maximum amount of greened vegetables which might be consumed daily. A daily dose of 100 grams of coppered peas or beans, which are the most highly coloured vegetables in the market, would not ordinarily contain more than 100 to 150 milligrams of copper. Such a bulk of greened vegetables is so large, however, that it would hardly be chosen as a part of a diet for many days in succession. Any amount of copper above 150 milligrams daily may therefore be considered excessive in practice. A small quantity is that amount which, in the ordinary use of vegetables, may be consumed over longer periods. From this point of view, 10 to 12 milligrams of copper may be regarded as the upper limit of a small quantity."

" It appears from our investigations that in certain directions even such small quantities of copper may have a deleterious action and must be considered injurious to health."

Other colouring matters in food. While in the past mineral matters definitely poisonous, such as lead chromate or arsenic compounds, have been used the colouring matters now employed are chiefly vegetable dyes and some aniline dyes which, so far as is known, have never caused food poisoning or disturbance. The Departmental Committee remarks " In regard to the colouring matters of modern origin, while we are of opinion that articles of food are very much preferable in their natural colours, we are unable to deduce from the evidence received that any injurious results have been traced to their consumption."

These colouring matters are a waste of material and cannot be considered necessary or desirable, while there is the possibility of their use in certain cases to mask the quality of food and to make saleable food which otherwise would be rejected as unfit for consumption or of inferior quality.

The actual Recommendations of this Departmental Committee were as follows:

"(a) That the use of formaldehyde or formalin, or preparations thereof, in foods or drinks be absolutely prohibited and that salicylic acid be not used in greater proportion than 1 grain per pint in liquid food and 1 grain per pound in solid food. Its presence in all cases to be declared.

"(b) That the use of any preservative or colouring matter whatever in milk offered for sale in the United Kingdom be constituted an offence under the Sale of Food and Drugs Acts.

"(c) That the only preservative which it shall be lawful to use in cream be boric acid or mixtures of boric acid and borax, and in amount not exceeding 0·25 per cent. expressed as boric acid. The amount of such preservative to be notified by a label upon the vessel.

"(d) That the only preservative to be used in butter and margarine be boric acid or mixtures of boric acid and borax, to be used in proportions not exceeding 0·5 per cent. expressed as boric acid.

"(e) That in the case of all dietetic preparations intended for the use of invalids or infants chemical preservatives of all kinds be prohibited.

"(f) That the use of copper salts in the so-called greening of preserved food be prohibited.

"(g) That means be provided, either by the establishment of a separate Court of Reference or by the imposition of more direct obligation on the Local Government Board, to exercise supervision over the use of preservatives and colouring matters in foods, and to prepare schedules of such as may be considered inimical to the public health."

There is general agreement amongst those entitled to hold an opinion in regard to conclusions (a), (b) and (e), while (c), (d) and (f) have a solid but not united body of scientific opinion behind them.

It is obvious that these Recommendations do not cover the ground but, while dealing with specific points, leave the use of preservatives in most substances still an open one. They do not recommend the compulsory recording of the presence of preservatives, do not state which preservatives may be used, or in what amounts, do not prohibit the sale of preservatives under fancy names. Even these Recommendations have not been made into laws.

It is important to realize the present inchoate condition of affairs in this country and that it is an extremely unsatisfactory one for all concerned, i.e. the general public, the food manufacturer and food vendor and the Local Authorities who have to administer the law.

The general public are prejudiced by, all unwittingly, being obliged to consume a considerable proportion of their food mixed with chemicals, the presence of which is unknown to the individual consumer and which many experts pronounce to be injurious. The consumer is given no opportunity to decline to buy such foods since the law does not require (except for cream) either their presence or their amount to be disclosed. He pays rates and taxes to be protected from injurious food, amongst other things, and he has no security that he gets what he pays for.

The food manufacturers and food vendors are in a position nearly as unsatisfactory. They do not know what steps they may take and what they may not do, to chemically preserve their commodities. A high standard of scrupulousness and regard for the possibly injurious action of preservatives may prejudice their business activities compared with trade rivals and competitors who lack their scruples, since the latter by a plentiful use of preservatives may avoid loss from damaged goods or the expenses of strict cleanliness in manufacture or storage. They are also subjected to inequalities of treatment, since in one area determined activity in dealing with preservatives may characterise the Local Authority, with consequent heavy legal expenses and burdensome litigation, while in another area the Local Authority regards the subject with complacency and no trouble is made.

Local Authorities and their officers are in an even more difficult position. Each case (with a few exceptions) in which preservatives are found has to be taken "on its merits." Costly legal machinery has to be evoked and each Local Authority has to be prepared (for they may not combine and pool legal actions), if they are attacking an industry which is united and provided with a strong financial backing, to take its case from Court to Court with ever-increasing expense to the rate-payer until an unchallengeable decision is given. For no branch of law do precedents so little govern the decisions, since conditions vary so widely in different cases, so there is small guarantee that in important cases decisions in the first Courts will be accepted as final.

That this is no fancy picture is shown by the very numerous instances in which cases are taken to the higher Courts and by the many instances in which the proceedings revolve round an unseemly wrangle between expert witnesses on the two sides repeating all the stock arguments and adducing the old experiments.

The Central Authority meanwhile largely repudiates all responsibility. It does not say which, if any, preservatives may be used or under what conditions or require their presence to be recorded. It appointed it is true a Departmental Committee, but it has not even legalised the few rather emasculated recommendations of that Committee. Its defenders may rejoin that the harmfulness of most of the preservatives used was not proved in the evidence taken by that Departmental Committee and that considerable divergence of opinion and of experimental results were manifested.

In the writer's opinion this attitude cannot be accepted as a sufficient or a satisfactory defence. The problem is difficult but not insoluble and it is for the State to take steps to solve it. *It is the duty of the State, as represented by the Controlling Department, to make up its mind as to preservatives in food*, and to embody it in the necessary legal form. Better to make it up wrongly in minor details than not to make it up at all. Cheaper to pay for the necessary investigations than to continue to squander money in fighting individual cases through the Courts. All this apart from the risk of serious injury to health from unregulated food dosing with chemicals.

If we had, as we have not at present, a proper Court of Scientific (Technical and Administrative) Experts to act as an advisory tribunal to a Ministry of Health it should be perfectly feasible to enact suitable regulations such as the following:

1. That no preservatives at all be permitted to be added to food, apart from salt, sugar and other stated substances, unless the fact is adequately stated on the label describing the food.

2. That the only preservatives which may be used are those contained in a government schedule, liable to revision from time to time.

3. That no preservatives may be sold for the preservation of food under fancy names and all must be vended in packages labelled with their full composition.

4. That the amounts of preservatives permitted to be added must not exceed in different articles the maximum amounts published in a schedule to be revised from time to time.

It is obvious that regulations of this nature imply a Government Department which is active not passive, positive not negative. They need not imply that sanctioned preservatives are harmless, merely that the evidence as to their injurious properties is insufficient to warrant their being excluded for the present.

The suggestion frequently advanced that the use of certain named preservatives should be prohibited by enactment is really rather a futile one, since the trade chemist will always be able to find new preservatives. The attitude should be that all must be prohibited until sanctioned and the State, as represented by its Health Ministry, should be courageous enough to make up its mind which to sanction, while being at the same time, on the one hand, always ready to withdraw its consent if the accumulated scientific data, which should be available and utilised as the result of that sanction, proves that any preservative is prejudicial, and on the other ready to admit the use of others which scientific evidence shows to be without detriment.

CHAPTER XIII

THE PREVENTION OF FOOD POISONING OUTBREAKS

IT has been shown in preceding chapters that while the majority of outbreaks of food infection and food poisoning are bacterial in origin a proportion are due to poisoning with chemical substances not derived from bacteria, such as arsenic or chemicals added to preserve food. Food poisoning from such wilful chemical additions or accidental contamination has been dealt with in Chapters XI and XII. Their prevention is largely a matter of more definite control over the addition of these substances by means of legal enactments restricting their wilful addition and of regulations exacting more care on the part of manufacturers as to the purity of substances to be added to articles to be used for human food. The need for such regulations and the form they should take has been sufficiently indicated in those chapters and further detailed consideration is not required.

The general problem of bacterial diseases transmitted by food considered in Chapter II is a very wide one and a complete discussion of methods of prevention would involve consideration of the question of the spread of all infectious diseases capable of being transmitted by food. These problems although introduced to complete the subject are really outside the scope of what is understood by food poisoning outbreaks.

The present chapter will therefore be confined to a discussion of the measures which are required, or which may be employed, to prevent the spread of bacterial food infections and food poisonings using these terms in the narrower limits which are usually applied to them in practical usage. The earlier chapters have shown that these conditions form a very definite group of outbreaks which are probably fairly common and it is of great importance to consider how far it is possible to limit their occurrence.

While recent bacteriological investigations have enormously widened our knowledge as to food poisoning and the distribution of the bacilli concerned, this increased knowledge has shown that the problem of prevention is far more difficult than was at one time supposed to be the case. In this it is comparable to the added administrative difficulties which have been caused by our increased knowledge as to the bacteriology and epidemiology of the acute infectious diseases.

It must be admitted that the prevention of food poisoning outbreaks is one of extreme difficulty.

If the original conception of food poisoning as due to the ingestion of food in a state of incipient decomposition had proved to be correct, prevention would have been a comparatively simple matter, resolving itself into steps to prevent this incipient decomposition and a careful instruction of the public as to the evil effects of tainted meat.

If the hypothesis which followed it—that these outbreaks were due to the consumption of the meat of animals suffering from certain specified diseases—had been shown to embrace the whole truth as to food poisoning, again preventive measures would not have been beyond satisfactory devising, consisting essentially as they would have done in a more rigid meat supervision and adequate punishment of those who neglected the statutory requirements as to traffic in such diseased food.

It has, however, been shown in the earlier sections that the first hypothesis is not in accord with modern knowledge, while the second is only a part of the truth.

From the review of existing knowledge given in the foregoing sections it is clear that, from the preventive standpoint, food poisoning cases must be looked upon as forming two groups:

(a) Those due to the consumption of meat derived from diseased animals. An *intra-vitam* infection with food poisoning bacilli, in most cases members of the Gaertner group, but probably occasionally with other varieties of bacteria.

(*b*) Those due to the contamination of healthy meat or other food with food poisoning bacilli derived from sources other than the food itself.

It is probable that the second group is considerably larger than the first.

The following preventive measures, general or direct, require careful consideration.

1. More exact knowledge of the subject amongst the medical profession generally.

It is evident that the knowledge of many general practitioners on this subject is antiquated and inaccurate. This is clear from a study of the medical evidence given at inquests upon cases of food poisoning. Death is usually ascribed to "ptomaine poisoning," the medical man explaining that under more or less unknown conditions food sometimes decomposes in the intestine with the formation of ptomaines which cause the symptoms. Surprise is frequently expressed that the meat showed no signs of being tainted. The term "ptomaine poisoning" given by the medical man as a full satisfactory and adequate explanation is accepted by the coroner and his jury as the whole of the matter and no further inquiry is deemed to be needed. It is, to say the least, unsatisfactory that there should be frequently such a discrepancy between medical evidence and readily ascertainable facts as to the causation of these cases. This has occurred, for example, in two outbreaks in which the writer had no difficulty in demonstrating that they were due to infection by Gaertner group bacilli. This *public* expression of views which are demonstrably wrong is not only damaging to the prestige of the medical profession as a scientific body but does more, it stifles inquiry and stops the elucidation of the truth.

The general medical and even public health textbooks are undoubtedly partly to blame as they still propound and accept theories of food poisoning which are inaccurate and retain a nomenclature which is misleading.

2. Detailed investigation of all food poisoning outbreaks.

It has been pointed out in earlier chapters that there are many lacunae in our knowledge as to the causes and channels of infection in food poisoning outbreaks. It must be accepted that many of these gaps would not exist if even that small proportion to the whole of outbreaks which are officially recognized were adequately investigated. The writer is particularly alive to this point as he has had the opportunity of studying the official reports of many scores of outbreaks recorded in this country. In a very large proportion of them scarcely anything was attempted in the direction of investigating the precise causation of the condition and the path of infection. In outbreak after outbreak all that was recorded was the details of the number of cases, the activities of the medical officer in putting a stop to it, a symposium as to the symptoms, a brief note as to the kind of food acting as the vehicle of spread, a note of surprise that the food appeared good, sometimes a description of the insanitary conditions which surrounded its preparation, but as regards investigations as to causation complete silence.

If the need for inquiry as to the method and paths of infection had been realized, if the realization had been followed by accurate investigation, it cannot be doubted that our knowledge of the means of prevention of this condition would have been immensely advanced.

Apart from these measures which really turn upon the neglect of this subject by the profession generally there are some definite preventive measures which at least merit consideration.

3. Meat inspection at the time of slaughter.

If an adequate and thorough system of meat inspection at the place of slaughter was in vogue in this country it would enable meat derived from animals suffering from infection with Gaertner group bacilli to be detected in many cases, and a certain number of food poisoning outbreaks would in this way be prevented.

Even with an adequate system, however, meat from such animals would continue to be passed in a number of instances, as in some cases the disease (enteritis, etc.) from which the animal was suffering might be overlooked. In several of the recorded continental outbreaks the meat was passed by the veterinary meat inspector, although it was subsequently ascertained that small lesions were present which were probably associated with the presence of the Gaertner group bacillus causing the outbreak.

There is indeed sometimes considerable difficulty in ascertaining how far Gaertner bacilli are likely to be present in some of the diseased conditions in animals associated with food poisoning. Bacteriological facilities should certainly be available to clear up doubtful cases but it is obviously impracticable to utilise bacteriology for the routine examination of all cases.

It may be concluded that while adequate supervision of meat at the time of slaughter will prevent some outbreaks it will not prevent more than a minority of them.

4. Separation of the slaughterhouse from food preparing places.

A careful study of the details of individual outbreaks as well as of theoretical considerations, shows that this is a most important preventive measure. In addition to the actual slaughtering, secondary procedures are frequently carried out in the slaughterhouse. The guts of pigs and other animals are not infrequently cleaned and washed in the slaughterhouse and then put in salt solution and used for sausage-casings. Brawn is also sometimes made and is frequently set to cool in the slaughterhouse.

From personal observations the writer finds that it is not at all uncommon for sausages to be made in the slaughterhouse and for the vessels containing the pickling fluid and meat in course of salting to be kept in the slaughterhouse. In none of the bye-laws which he has seen has there been any clause prohibiting such practices, nor are they prohibited in the model bye-laws.

This is a most important matter. It is evident that animals

may recover from Gaertner infections, either completely or sufficiently for their carcases to be passed as satisfactory by the butcher and yet such animals may harbour living virulent bacilli of this group in the spleen or other organs or in the intestinal contents. If in the same slaughterhouse prepared foods are made or stored, infection of these foods is invited, and undoubtedly in this way a number of food poisoning outbreaks have originated.

5. Enforcement of a higher standard of cleanliness in premises where made-up meat foods are prepared.

The most striking fact which emerges from the study of any series of meat poisoning outbreaks is the very large number of cases in which the vehicle of infection has been brawn, meat pies, sausages or other form of made-up meat. Investigation of the condition of the premises and the actual procedures practised has almost invariably shown that, speaking generally, cleanliness was not practised in the preparation of these materials nor were the premises of such a kind as would enable cleanliness and avoidance of contamination to be secured. Definite opportunities for excretal contamination of the food, during preparation or subsequently, were usually present.

Existing powers with regard to foodstuffs urgently need revision in many directions, but in nothing do they require strengthening more than in connection with the preparation of made-up meat foods.

Take, for example, a substance like brawn. In making it its constituents are heated so that competing bacilli are largely eliminated. When finished it constitutes a most favourable nutrient material for bacilli, with abundance of jelly, etc. This culture medium is set to cool, and usually cools slowly, so that over many hours it is maintained at temperatures which greatly favour bacterial multiplication. Frequently in practice the brawn is set to cool in places which necessitate its bacterial contamination, and sometimes it is put in places, such as slaughterhouses, were specific dangerous bacterial contamination is likely to occur. The brawn maker can do this quite unchecked by the supervision

of the Local Sanitary Authority. He has neither to license
nor to register his premises or himself and is not subject to
any supervision by the Local Authority, apart from their
general powers in regard to food inspection.

The anomaly of the existing legal position is apparent if
these non-existent powers are compared with the comparative stringent regulations governing the preparation of bread
and its supervision. Bread is a substance which is a quite
unimportant source of bacterial infection and the amount
which does occur (i.e. from dirty handling of loaves) is largely
independent of the supervision exercised. As potential
vehicles for the spread of disease made foods are vastly more
important than bread.

A proper system of bye-laws and licensing of all premises
upon which made-up meat foods are prepared are required
and would be of material importance in limiting food poisoning outbreaks.

6. The limitation of diseases in animals caused by bacilli of the Gaertner group.

It has been shown in Chapter VI (including Addendum II)
that there are many pathological conditions in animals due
to infection with bacilli of the Gaertner group or in which
these organisms are present as secondary invaders. In
Chapter X it was explained that the hypothesis which best
accounts for the causation of the majority of outbreaks is
that the bacilli are derived from animals which are either at
the time suffering from disease due to Gaertner group bacilli
or acting as carriers of these bacilli.

Looking beyond the immediate steps required to prevent
the infection of food for human consumption, it follows as
an important practical inference that any steps which can
be taken to limit the prevalence of these diseases in animals
will diminish the chances of specific infection of human food
and so will tend to lessen the number of food poisoning outbreaks.

Such a limitation of the amount of animal Gaertner disease
is a difficult matter to secure but is not beyond the range

of practicability. Combined veterinary and bacteriological investigation should be made as to the extent to which Gaertner group diseases in animals occur in this country and how far the bacilli persist in a virulent condition in animals which have recovered from acute attacks. The data mentioned in Chapter X make it probable that in certain cases they may persist for considerable periods.

In this connection it may be doubted how far it is wise, or indeed justifiable, to distribute broadcast without any check or supervision innumerable Gaertner group bacilli in the form of the various rat and mice viruses, for the purpose of destroying these rodents. These bacilli differ in no particular except virulence from the Gaertner group bacilli associated with food poisoning outbreaks, and while it is advanced that they are not pathogenic to man (and numerous instances of their free use without harm favour this contention), there are many instances in which cases or groups of cases of illness in man have been attributed to infection from these viruses.

One prominent characteristic of the Gaertner group of organisms is their varying virulence, and we are not in a position to negative the possibility that strains, originally non-virulent to man, may, by single or repeated passage through rats or mice, acquire a virulence sufficient to enable them to infect man, either directly or indirectly, by causing disease in the animals used for human consumption.

The danger of contamination of food by excreta of rats has been dealt with in Chapter X, p. 176.

7. Steps to obtain official cognisance of food poisoning outbreaks.

There is not the slightest doubt that a very large number of cases, and even considerable outbreaks, of food poisoning and food infection pass unrecognised by the official authorities, and remain unrecorded, uninvestigated and sometimes unrecognised.

As illustrating how slender the chances may be of such cases coming to light the outbreak at Bristol in 1909 (quoted by the writer in his Report to the Local Government Board) may be mentioned.

No less than fifty-four known cases are recorded, but all of them were ill four days before it came to the notice of the health authorities. This information was purely fortuitous, as it was only obtained through one of the office staff reporting that his wife and neighbours were all suffering. It is reasonably certain that if an employee had not been affected the Health Department would have known nothing about it.

If adequate measures are to be taken to prevent the frequent occurrence of food poisoning outbreaks, it is essential that all outbreaks, however small, should be brought to the knowledge of the medical officer of health and be thoroughly studied by him, with the assistance at an early stage of a bacteriologist. The excellent memorandum of the Local Government Board dated September, 1911, on the investigation of outbreaks of illness suspected to be due to food poisoning, indicates the lines on which such inquiries should be conducted and has served a valuable purpose in stimulating interest and insuring the investigation of many outbreaks brought to the notice of the medical officer of health.

A further question is how is this official cognizance to be obtained. It might be suggested that this group of cases should be added to the list of diseases which have to be notified by medical men to the medical officer of health. There are, however, considerable objections to this course, such as the fact that a medical man is not consulted in all cases and that the obscurities of definition as to what is included in the term would in practice lead to difficulties. All kinds of trivial cases might have to be investigated. It is, however, highly desirable that more co-operation between medical practioners and medical officers of health should obtain as regards the unofficial notification and investigation of such cases. This would be facilitated if the services of a bacteriologist were always available free of charge to medical practitioners, through the medical officer of health, to examine material from possible or actual cases.

More could also be done by the education of the public,

inducing them to look more to their Health Department for advice and help. The average citizen looks upon the sanitary service for which he pays as a penal and detective organization of narrow scope rather than as an advisory body with extensive and wide functions. Usually when food poisoning cases have resulted the survivors and their relations are convinced that someone is very much to blame and the target of their animosity is, as a rule, the food vendor. It should be equally natural for them also to take the matter to their Health Department for explanation and advice. In this way many outbreaks would come to light and the appropriate steps be taken to limit and study them.

CHAPTER XIV

METHODS OF INVESTIGATION OF FOOD POISONING OUTBREAKS

IT will be evident from preceding chapters that outbreaks of food poisoning may be of different kinds and that the exact methods of investigation required will vary according to the nature of the outbreak. Outbreaks of infectious diseases (such as typhoid fever) spread by food, although discussed in Chapter II to complete the subject, do not really come under the definition, as ordinarily understood, of attacks of food poisoning and need not be further considered in this chapter. The interesting cases of food idiosyncrasy are obvious from their nature and do not give rise to outbreaks. The cases which have to be considered group themselves under attacks of poisoning or gastro-intestinal disease from inherently poisonous foods, from foods bacterially contaminated and from foods impregnated with poisonous chemical substances. Of these the group due to contamination of the food by specific bacilli is by far the largest and most important.

Considerable difficulty is often experienced in obtaining particulars and in numerous instances even extensive outbreaks never come to the notice of the authorities. This difficulty is increased when the cases implicated are not confined to the area of the one local authority. This is particularly likely to occur when a food, such as cheese or tinned meat, is part of a large consignment only a portion of which is affected and in which the good and the infected samples have been distributed impartially over a wide area. It is particularly important in such cases that the Central Health Authority (the Ministry of Health) should be promptly consulted and its machinery utilized to make the necessary inquiries in other areas. The Central Authority is also in a position to make detailed inquiries and investigations at the place of origin of the food, a procedure which is frequently very difficult for the Local Authority to undertake.

An outbreak in 1910 will serve as a good example of the necessity and value of thoroughly following up inquiries. The first cases were reported at St Helens in August, 1910, when thirty-two persons were attacked. In the same month there were twenty-one cases at Carlisle. Further investigation by the Local Government Board elicited six cases in Gateshead in September and fifteen in November at Hessle. In every instance the outbreak was associated with the consumption of the meat from a six pound tin of a particular brand of corned beef, one can only being implicated in each instance. The short incubation period and other features showed that the outbreak was due to bacterial toxins, but their nature was not ascertained. It was evident that a certain but unknown proportion of a particular consignment, a very large one of several million pounds of meat, was infected and the firm in question with considerable public spirit agreed to stop the sale of the whole of the consignment remaining unsold. This satisfactory determination of a difficult problem would not have been reached without the active co-operation of the Central Department and the extensive inquiries which they instituted.

The investigation of outbreaks is dealt with in a clear and valuable Report issued by the Local Government Board (1911), which should be consulted by every medical officer of health.

I. Inquiries to be instituted.

Information usually reaches the medical officer of health, or other member of the Health Department, in the form that a number of persons have suffered, within a short period, from gastro-intestinal symptoms with acute onset. This information may be received from one or more of the sufferers or their friends, from local medical practitioners, or, not at all infrequently, the first information is that a fatal case of this type of unknown origin has occurred. If anything like an adequate investigation is to be made it is imperative that the inquiries should be prompt and thorough.

The following investigations are always necessary:

(a) *An attempt to secure a complete list of the cases.* Obtained by

(1) An inquiry at the homes of the known infected households. This will probably lead to a special article of food being suspected.

(2) Inquiries of medical practitioners as to similar cases of illness, each of them serving as a fresh centre of investigation.

(3) In certain cases it may be necessary to make house to house inquiries in the implicated area.

(4) If the outbreak is extensive the medical officers of health of adjacent or implicated areas should be consulted.

(b) *Detailed particulars of the individual cases of illness.* The details required are:

Clinical features.

Exact date and time the food was consumed.

Quantity of affected food eaten by each person.

Interval since eating and onset of symptoms.

(c) *Evidence as to the vehicle of infection.* As a rule the initial inquiries have clearly demonstrated the particular food implicated, but if this is not the case the investigation would have to include an intimate study of the food consumed by the sufferers and by those in the same households who escaped. Sometimes the investigation has to be carried a stage further and the particular ingredients in a composite food studied (e.g. the meat and gravy separately in a meat pie) to ascertain the exact article infected.

(d) *A detailed study of the history of the implicated food.* These must include

Precise nature of the implicated food.

If compounded the different ingredients and by whom mixed and prepared.

The source of the food traced back to the animal itself (if of animal origin). Size of the consignment and fate of the rest of the batch.

Particulars as to any treatment or preparation of the food before consumption and by whom carried out.

How far the particular food was fully or inadequately cooked.

In every case the dates of purchase and of any domestic treatment should be ascertained and recorded.

These inquiries must be instituted both in the homes of the sufferers and at the places of preparation.

Details as to the extent to which the food presented abnormalities of taste, smell or appearance, during its different stages are occasionally of importance.

(*e*) *Evidence as to the source of infection of the food.* This is the part of the inquiry which is so habitually neglected but which merits the closest attention if progress is to be achieved in regard to the prevention of outbreaks.

In some outbreaks—for example, those of a chemical nature—this may be a simple matter but in the more common bacterial types most painstaking inquiries, associated with bacteriological examination, may be required to elucidate the source and paths of infection.

Points requiring particular attention are

(1) The sanitary conditions under which the food was made, prepared for consumption, cooled or stored. In particular any opportunities for specific contamination must be looked for, such as gut scraping or other association with animal excreta or contamination from rats and mice.

(2) If the food is of animal origin (meat or milk) inquiries should be made as to evidence of healthiness or illness of the animals supplying, at the time of or before slaughter, or amongst others of the same herd.

Note. The price at which sold may throw indirectly light upon this matter.

(3) The possibility of the infection being from a human carrier. Evidence of illness amongst those who handled the food. This inquiry is greatly facilitated by bacteriological examinations.

II. Collection of material.

It is obviously of importance that this should be obtained at the earliest time possible after the onset of the outbreak. A full investigation will comprise the examinations set out below, but as frequently not all the material will be obtainable it is worth emphasising that a fairly complete elucidation of the cause of the outbreak may be obtainable when only comparatively slender material is available for examination.

(*A*) *Nature of material to examine.*

(1) *Portions of the actual food consumed.* This is frequently unobtainable, particularly in limited outbreaks. Obviously much depends upon the interval between the onset and the inquiry. If food is sent for examination care should be taken to indicate if it is part of the same food as was actually consumed by sufferers or if merely a sample of food of similar origin. A good many of the blank results obtained undoubtedly have been due to the food sent being the latter and not actually infected food at all.

If doubt exists as to which ingredient is implicated in a composite food, samples of the separate components should be obtained.

(2) *Materials from fatal cases.* If available this is by far the most valuable material for investigation. The samples to be transmitted should be spleen, liver (part is sufficient), part of a bone containing bone marrow, heart blood in a sterile bottle or in the unopened heart, piece of small intestine (ligatured), stomach (ligatured) with unopened contents. Other organs such as the kidneys may be included but are not really necessary.

(3) *Materials from living cases.* Samples of blood (from finger or ear) for agglutination tests should be collected and transmitted in the ordinary way (in sealed glass pipettes) from as many cases as possible. These specimens should not be collected at the onset of the illness as specific agglutinins will hardly have had time to be produced. They are of particular value when other sources of material are not available, since they yield positive results in Gaertner infections for a considerable period after the outbreak has subsided.

If chemical or mushroom poisoning is suspected vomited materials should be sent for examination, if obtainable.

Dejecta specimens are of value, particularly when there are no samples available from fatal cases. They are more difficult to examine and negative results are of little significance. They should be sent as fresh as possible.

(4) *Materials from infected animals.* These are only required in special cases and whether they are needed or not arises at a later stage out of the results of the preliminary investigations.

They may include the examination of milk, blood, dejecta and discharges of different animals.

A good example of the value of such examinations is given on p. 162 in connection with a milk spread outbreak.

(B) *Methods of transmission.*

The examinations required are almost invariably bacteriological and the most satisfactory plan is to arrange with the bacteriologist for him to send the sterile bottles, jars, pipettes, etc., required, so that the material may be transmitted with proper precautions and under suitable conditions. If samples are likely to be delayed in transit they should be sent in ice-boxes.

Sometimes there is no time to communicate first with the bacteriologist and obtain outfits from him. In such cases the following note by Durham (1898) on an emergency outfit may be useful:

"*Impromptu method of making a simple freezing apparatus.* Take a moderately large tin, such as a biscuit tin, and a wooden box of sufficient size to give three or four inches clear space in every direction when the tin is placed within it. Put a layer of sawdust three or four inches deep at the bottom; stand the tin upon this, and fill the surrounding space with sawdust also. The various organs, after being removed with as much cleanliness as possible, are each wrapped in a clean cloth, wetted (not wringing wet) with $1:500$ $HgCl_2$, and further wrapped and sealed, each separately in a piece of gutta-percha tissue (most easily done with a trace of chloroform); they are then put into one or more watertight tins (those $\frac{1}{4}$ or $\frac{1}{2}$ lb. tins in which some tobacco is sent out are admirable, they may be more securely closed by means of a paraffin candle and a warm poker). The tobacco tins are placed within the larger tin, together with pounded ice and common salt, in the proportion of 3 lbs. of ice to 1 lb. of salt. The lid is placed on the larger tin, and the wooden outer box filled up with sawdust. An apparatus which holds the above quantities of ice and salt will keep about ½ pint hard frozen for more than twenty-four hours. There can be no difficulty in obtaining these materials at a moment's notice."

III. Laboratory investigations.

The scientific and practical value of the investigation of very many outbreaks has been spoilt owing to the suspected food being sent for chemical examination under the dominance of the fallacious "ptomaine" hypothesis. Naturally the analyst finds no ptomaines and the examination of important material is wasted. Chemical examinations may be required in special cases, but they are *special* cases and in all but a tiny minority of cases the material should be sent to a bacteriologist for examination. If the possibility of chemical poisoning has not been eliminated the bacteriologist should be asked to retain some of the material for subsequent chemical analysis, and this can usually be done without detriment since most of the chemical substances possible as causes of food poisoning are stable bodies and will not decompose or spoil by being kept awhile in the ice chest.

Bacteriological and pathological examinations.

(a) *The suspected foodstuffs.* The precise methods of examination will vary slightly with the nature of the food, but should be on the following lines:

The physical appearance, smell and chemical reaction should be noted carefully. Any deviations from the natural appearance of normal food of the kind under examination should be recorded. Aerobic and anaerobic cultivations, feeding and inoculation tests may all have to be made.

Cultural examinations. It is important to obtain a uniform and characteristic sample. This can be conveniently done by mixing up selected portions with sterile instruments and adding to sterile water in a stoppered bottle, mixing thoroughly. If a quantitative examination is to be made a definite quantity of food must be added to a definite quantity of water. A fairly complete examination would include examination for Gaertner group bacilli, *proteus* group bacilli, *B. coli* and allied organisms, and for anaerobic bacilli such as *B. botulinus* and the putrefactive anaerobes.

The most reliable method, in the writer's opinion, to isolate Gaertner group bacilli is to brush some of the emulsion directly over a series of lactose-salicin-saccharose neutral red bile salt agar (L.S.S.B.A.) and to add also some of the emulsion to dulcite malachite green broth tubes (for composition of these and other media see Addendum VI). After twelve to eighteen hours incubation the latter, suitably diluted, is brushed over a few L.S.S.B.A. plates. This broth medium favours the growth of Gaertner group bacilli over the other intestinal bacteria. The addition of the salicin and saccharose eliminates those para-Gaertner organisms which ferment these substances.

All the white colonies (at least on the primary plates) must be investigated. This is most rapidly done by agglutination tests with powerful *B. enteritidis* and *B. aertrycke* sera. For this preliminary sorting the most convenient plan is to use sera with a titre of not less than 1 : 1000. A dilution of 1 : 100 is prepared of each of these two sera and a loopful of each is placed on a series of coverslips, one loopful of each in separate drops. The white colonies are all previously numbered. With a sterile platinum needle a *trace* of colony No. 1 is added to each of the two loopfuls on the one coverglass. The latter is everted and fixed with vaseline over a hanging drop slide in the ordinary way and the colony number and time marked on the slide with a glass pencil. If the orientation of the two drops is kept the same throughout, the sera used need not be marked on the slide. The other colonies are similarly treated and in this way a large number of hanging drop preparations can be put up in a short time. When the serum dilution is only to about one-tenth of the titre as recommended a time interval of fifteen minutes at room temperature is long enough. The hanging drop preparations are examined microscopically and those showing no agglutination rejected. Those showing definite clumping with either serum are culturally worked out and accurate agglutination tests made. This procedure will very rapidly eliminate the great majority of colonies not of the Gaertner group, but it is important to remember that the reacting colonies cannot be accepted without further tests as Gaertner organisms. It is merely a rapid method of sorting out the colonies worth investigating.

The cultural characters of the true Gaertner organisms are given in Chapter VI, but for the convenience of workers it may be said that perhaps the simplest and quickest plan is to inoculate each of the selected colonies into six media: i.e. gelatine slope, litmus milk, peptone water, dulcite litmus broth, glucose litmus broth, salicin + saccharose + lactose litmus broth (the last three in double tubes). The other two important fermentation tests with raffinose and mannite need only be applied later to confirm. Motility and microscopic appearance must of course be ascertained, the gelatine slope culture being convenient for this purpose.

The agglutination tests must be taken to the limit of agglutination. In important cases it may be necessary to immunize a rabbit with the isolated strain before a definite opinion as to the sub-group is given. Absorption tests also may be required.

The presence of *B. coli* group organisms in the food can be judged from the number of red colonies on the modified L.S.S.B.A. plates.

B. proteus isolation. The writer has experimented extensively with many different forms of media, with or without aniline dyes, for this purpose but has not up to the present obtained a medium which can be considered satisfactory. Two methods may be tried:

(i) Direct plating of a suitably diluted emulsion of the medium over a series of 10 per cent. gelatine plates. Not less than three in series should be used as the extent of bacterial contamination is usually very problematical. The plates, incubated at 21° C., are examined after twenty-four, thirty and forty-eight hours respectively for the fairly characteristic liquefying colonies of *Proteus vulgaris* and for the non-liquefying colonies of *Proteus zenkeri* with their characteristic thread-like processes spreading through the medium. Possible colonies should be sub-cultivated into broth, replated to

ensure purity (a very necessary precaution) and worked out
culturally.

(ii) Method of Choukevitch (1911). A little of the material
for examination is added to the lower part of a tube of
sloped agar, great care being taken to inoculate only the
very bottom of the medium. The tube is incubated for
twenty-four to thirty-six hours. If *B. proteus* is present it is
supposed to extend up to the upper part of the agar and be
present there in pure culture. As a subsidiary method to
determine if *B. proteus* (using the term for the group) is
present the writer has found this method of value and sometimes has been able to isolate organisms of this group by
its means, when failure resulted with other methods.

It may be mentioned that *B. proteus* organisms can also be
isolated sometimes from lactose bile salt neutral red agar
plates, these organisms growing as white circular colonies.

The examination of the foodstuff for the ordinary anaerobes
is not of much service, as if found their presence is of no
significance. If the symptoms suggest botulism *B. botulinus*
may be specially looked for, while its absence can be more
definitely ascertained by inoculation tests.

If *B. botulinus* is present the foodstuff will probably have
a distinct butyric acid smell. If the subcutaneous injection
of a watery extract of the suspected material into a rabbit
fails to reproduce the characteristic symptoms of botulism
in animals (see p. 152) it can be assumed that the toxins of
B. botulinus are absent and cultural tests are hardly necessary.

The methods for the isolation of anaerobes have been
materially improved during the last few years. For the
isolation of *B. botulinus* and other anaerobes the plate
method of Wilson is useful, while the method of eliminating
the oxygen by using palladium or platinum asbestos to
combine it with hydrogen is very convenient. For an excellent account of these more modern methods see Fildes
(1917).

Since the spores of *B. botulinus* are not highly resistant
the method of heating to 80° C. for ten to fifteen minutes to
eliminate non-sporing forms should not be employed. A

watery emulsion of the material for examination should be spread over glucose serum-agar plates grown anaerobically, while other portions of the emulsion are added to glucose meat broth tubes and incubated anaerobically for several days and then plated on glucose-agar. The temperature of incubation should be 20–22° C. The characters of this bacillus are described in Chapter IX.

(b) *Material from human cases.* The examination of material from autopsies is conducted in a similar manner but is usually much easier, the bacilli being frequently present in pure or nearly pure culture. Only a few L.S.S.B.A. and other plates need to be inoculated from each organ. Frequently the presence of Gaertner group bacilli can be determined within twenty-four hours.

The examination of the contents of the intestine or of excreta specimens is a more troublesome business and a considerable number of plates must be made, while enrichment methods should also be employed. The white colonies on the plates should be sorted out with the Gaertner group sera as recommended for the examination of the foodstuff. If the examination of the excreta is at all delayed, as is usually the case, Gaertner bacilli may be very scanty and hard to isolate.

The testing of the agglutinative properties of the blood of actual or suspected cases is a very important part of the investigation, since, as already mentioned, even when no other material at all is available for examination it sometimes is sufficient to determine accurately the cause of infection.

The sera should be tested against stock cultures of all three strains of the Gaertner group, *B. enteritidis*, *B. suipestifer* (*aertrycke*) and *B. paratyphosus B.* Dilutions of 1 in 30 and 1 in 100 may be conveniently employed as a routine. If positive then 1 : 300, 1 : 500, etc., should be tested, if necessary to the limit of agglutination. Some of the serum should be reserved, or fresh specimens taken, to test against any Gaertner group bacilli isolated from the food or from post mortem material.

A pathological examination of the organs from fatal cases

yield little or nothing of practical value and is not of much importance.·

(c) *Material from affected animals.* This will vary with the nature of the material to be examined, but will be on the same lines as material from human cases.

In regard to testing the agglutinative properties of sera from animals it should be mentioned that caution is necessary in their interpretation, since quite healthy animals may give positive findings to a certain extent (see p. 87).

Chemical examination.

(a) *Examination for ptomaines.* As explained this is rarely required but special circumstances may make it advisable to test for these bodies if only to demonstrate their absence. For this purpose Brieger's method as described in Dixon-Mann's *Forensic Medicine* (1908, p. 678) may be employed: "An alcoholic extract obtained from the organic matter which contains the ptomaine is precipitated with neutral lead acetate (in order to remove amorphous albuminoid and other inert matter), filtered, and the filtrate evaporated to a small bulk; the residue is dissolved in water through which H_2S is passed until the lead is thrown down. After filtration the solution is evaporated to a syrup, which, when cold, is extracted with alcohol, and the filtered extract precipitated with an alcoholic solution of $HgCl_2$. Advantage is taken of the varying solubility of the double salts formed by ptomaines with mercuric chloride to effect their separation by treatment with boiling water. The solutions thus obtained are severally decomposed by H_2S and, after removal of the mercurous sulphide, are evaporated down so as to cause the ptomaine salts to crystallise out. Further separation is accomplished by forming double salts of the ptomaines with $PtCl_4$ and $AuCl_3$. During the various processes, especially in the early ones, the temperature should not exceed 40° C., nor should the solutions be allowed to acquire more than a feebly acid reaction."

"As free bases ptomaines are mostly liquid; some are crystallisable; some are volatile, others are not; they form salts more or less easily crystallisable. Like vegetable alkaloids, ptomaines are precipitated by most of the alkaloidal group-tests."

Their toxicity should be tested by injection and feeding of animals (guinea-pigs, rabbits, kittens), while if necessary chemical tests for individual ptomaines may be employed (see Vaughan and Novy).

(b) *Examination for evidence of putrefactive changes.* The chemical tests for early decomposition changes in meat foods mentioned in the textbooks are really useless as they are unreliable and only definite when the meat is obviously putrefactive by smell and appearance. The writer with Mr D. Wood has spent much time in investigating the practicability of other chemical tests but up to the present the results are not sufficiently advanced to be worth reproducing.

(c) *Examination for poisonous metals.* The metals which may have to be looked for are set out in Chapter XI. Suitable tests and methods of estimation will be found in Analytical Textbooks. While fairly simple to detect their estimation is a matter of considerable experience and should be left to the expert chemist, and to describe the methods in detail would occupy space which is unnecessary, in view of the excellent available descriptions.

(d) *Examination for preservatives.* As for (c) it is not proposed to give here the different tests and methods of estimation. The latter require considerable experience.

It is important to remember that occasionally preservatives are present in amount sufficient to retard bacterial growth and so, if their presence is not suspected, give a false idea of bacterial purity.

REFERENCES (including Addendum VI).

Bierotte and Machida (1910). *Münch. med. Woch.* LVII. 636.
Cary (1916). *Am. Journ. of Public Health*, VI. 124.
Choukevitch (1911). *Ann. de l'Inst Pasteur*, XXV. 852.
Conradi (1909). *Zeit. f. Fleisch- und Milch-hyg.* 341.
Durham (1898). *Brit. Med. Journ.* II. 1801.
Fildes (1917). "Methods for cultivating the anaerobic bacteria,"
    Special Report, No. 12, Medical Research Committee.
Filenski (1915). *Arb. a. d. Kais. Gesund.* L. 133.

Horn (1910). *Zeit. f. Infekt. der Haustiere*, VIII. 424.

Local Government Board. Memorandum on the investigation of outbreaks of illness suspected to be due to food poisoning, September, 1911.

Metzner (1910). *Tierärztl. Zentralb.* 436.

Müller (1910). *Centralb. f. Bakt.* 1 Abt. Orig. LVI 277.

Savage (1908). *Journ. Roy. San. Inst.* XXIX. 366.

—— (1918). *Journ. of Hyg.* XVII. 34.

Slooten (1909). *Centralb. f. Bakt.* 1 Abt. Ref. XLIII. 193.

Vaughan and Novy (1903). *Cellular Toxins.*

Weinzirl and Newton (1914). *Am. Journ. of Public Health*, IV. 413.

Zweifel (1911). *Centralb. f. Bakt.* 1 Abt. Orig. LVIII. 115.

Zwick and Weichel (1911). *Arb. a. d. Kais. Gesund.* XXVIII. 327.

ADDENDUM VI.

I. DIFFERENTIATION OF THE TYPHOID-COLON GROUP.

In the main this is based upon fermentation tests. The following arboreal
statement may be convenient for reference:

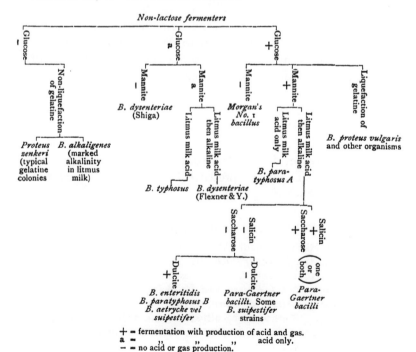

$+$ = fermentation with production of acid and gas.
a =   ,,   ,,   ,,   acid only.
$-$ = no acid or gas production.

The most convenient substances to quickly differentiate the main groups are lactose, glucose, mannite and litmus milk. Lactose differentiates at once between the B. *coli* group (lactose fermenters) and the rest—the non-lactose fermenters

NOTE. This statement does not mean that the tests given are sufficient to establish the identification of the types mentioned. Of course all the essential characters of the strain have to be determined. All that is intended to be shown is a convenient means of rapidly sorting out the organisms studied into their possible groups, leaving it for other and confirmatory tests to complete the diagnosis. There are probably, in addition, a considerable number of non-pathogenic and unnamed lactose fermenters which closely simulate some of the above types.

II. THE BACTERIAL CONTENT OF ORDINARY MEAT FOODS.

Many mistakes have been made by bacteriologists through an inadequate acquaintance with normal conditions and the presence of particular bacteria given an unwarranted significance owing to a failure to recognize that the conditions found were in no way special but were those found normally, or but quantitatively exaggerated, under ordinary practical conditions. This being the case it may be of value to append a few particulars as to actual findings in meat foods under ordinary conditions and quite unassociated with outbreaks of food poisoning or other evidence of harmful properties.

A. Internal organs of food producing animals. The question as to how far these organs are sterile has been investigated by a number of workers. Conradi (1909) using a special enrichment method found bacteria on seventy-two occasions out of 162 organs from 150 healthy animals. Of these bacteria thirty were anaerobic, forty-two aerobic. The aerobic organisms included B. *coli*, B. *lactis aerogenes*, streptococci, etc., while the anaerobes were chiefly of the butyric acid group.

Bierotte and Machida (1910) employed a modified Conradi method and obtained very similar results. They examined fifty-four organs from eleven quite healthy animals and found bacilli in thirty-two.

Zwick and Weichel (1911) also found bacteria in the internal organs in a number of cases.

The writer (Savage, 1918) examined the spleens of twenty-four pigs and ten calves, all within a few hours of death, for aerobic bacilli. Exactly half of the pig and half of the calf spleens were sterile, the remaining 50 per cent. containing bacilli which were not completely identified but were mostly B. *coli*, non-lactose fermenters allied to B. *coli*, streptococci and staphylococci. No special enrichment methods were used in these examinations.

These investigations show that the presence of organisms in the internal organs of domestic animals, even when examined within a few hours of death, does not of necessity indicate that they have any pathological relationship.

B. Fresh musculature. Gaertner in 1908 found that bacilli were present on the surface of fresh meat but had not penetrated, if the examination was made within three days of slaughter, while by the end of ten days they had not penetrated more than 0·5 inch into the interior. These results were confirmed by Foster (1908) as regards the general sterility of the interior of fresh meat.

Horn (1910) found bacteria in the interior of the musculature finding, as might be expected, that the number varied with the time since slaughter.

Conradi, also Meyer and Rommeler, found bacteria in a certain proportion of cases. Metzner (1910) investigated 145 cases and found the meat free from aerobic bacteria, but did not examine for anaerobic organisms. Also Junach, Grabert and Mergell are quoted by Filenski (1915) as finding the flesh of slaughtered animals sterile (the original references are not available).

Müller (1910) in 46 per cent. of investigated cases found bacteria present.

Anyone who takes the trouble to prepare and stain microscopic preparations from the surface of even quite fresh meat will be able to demonstrate the presence of large numbers of bacteria. With the interval since slaughter the numbers increase very rapidly and after 20–24 hours they are very numerous. Also when sections are cut and stained they can be seen penetrating between the muscle fibres.

The question as to how far perfectly fresh unhandled meat is sterile would appear to be undecided from the above discrepant findings.

C. Chopped meat ("hackfleisch"). Zweifel (1911) at Leipzig examined 248 specimens of "hackfleisch" obtained quite fresh and in 165 cases found *B. proteus* and other bacilli, all non-pathogenic to mice by feeding.

Weinzirl and Newton (1914) examined what they call Hamburger steak, which is really scraps of meat collected during the day from the trimmings of steaks, etc. They found the number of bacteria, in the forty-four samples examined, to vary from 270,000 to 88 millions per gramme. All but two would be passed by physical tests (smell, appearance, etc.). The numbers of bacteria present were naturally much higher in warm weather. They suggested a standard of ten million bacteria per gramme as the limit.

It is obvious that with meat of this kind the number of bacteria present will vary directly with the degree and cleanliness of the handling, the time since killing and the prevailing temperature.

D. Sausages. The writer (Savage, 1908) obtained the following figures from twenty-seven sausage samples, all examined the same day as prepared and all obtained from different sources.

B. coli organisms			No. of specimens
Less than 10 per grm. of sausage meat			0
10—100 ,, ,, ,,			4
100—1000 ,, ,, ,,			6
1000—10,000 ,, ,, ,,			4
10,000—100,000 ,, ,, ,,			7
Over 100,000 ,, ,, ,,			2
Over 100,000 but actual number not estimated			4

The number of organisms present was determined for a few of the samples and varied from 360,000 to over 600,000 per gramme. Streptococci were also present in large numbers in a majority of the samples examined.

Slooten (1909) with sausage of various ages found up to one million bacteria per gramme of sausage.

Cary (1916) examined thirty-four pork sausages from Chicago shops. All but four contained *B. coli*, while 64 per cent. contained over 100 *B. coli* per gramme of meat. The average bacterial content was 158,000 per grm. growing at 37° C. (2500 to 1,538,000 as extremes), and 9,018,000 at 20° C. (650 to 200,000,000 as extremes). Cary found *Proteus vulgaris* in three out of seven samples of scrapings from sausage casings, while this organism was isolated eleven times (33 per cent.) from the sausages themselves.

E. Brawn. Brawn is, or should be, thoroughly boiled when prepared so that whatever its original bacterial contamination it should be free from *B. coli* and non-sporing bacteria when made. As a rule this is the case, but brawn is a material very favourable to bacterial multiplication, so that if, after preparation, it is placed in positions liable to bacterial contamination specimens will soon show a high bacterial content.

Of eleven samples examined by the writer *B. coli* was absent in 0·1 grm. in seven, present 1–10 per grm. in one, present 5000–10,000 in one, while in the remaining samples these organisms were about 50,000 per grm.

III.   COMPOSITION OF SOME OF THE MEDIA RECOMMENDED.

A. Lactose-salicin-saccharose neutral red bile salt agar (L.S.S.B.A.). Sodium taurocholate 5 grammes, Witte's (or other suitable) peptone 20 grammes, and distilled water 1 litre, are boiled up together, 20 grammes of agar are added and dissolved in the solution in the autoclave in the ordinary way. The medium is cleared with white of egg and filtered. After filtration, 10 grammes each of lactose, saccharose and salicin and 5 c.c. of recently prepared 1 per cent. neutral red solution are added. The medium is then tubed, or put into small flasks, and sterilized for fifteen minutes on three successive days.

B. Dulcite malachite green broth. Liebig's extract 10 grammes, peptone 10 grammes, sodium chloride 5 grammes, are boiled up with a litre of distilled water. The mixture, after filtration, is made up accurately to a +1 per cent. reaction, and 5 grammes of dulcite are added; 0·5 gramme of powdered malachite green is very accurately weighed out and also added. The mixture, usually slightly turbid, is steamed for thirty minutes, and again filtered. It is tubed, 10 c.c. into each tube, and sterilized for thirty minutes on two successive days.

If dulcite is not readily obtainable it may be replaced by glucose, but dulcite is preferable.

C. Serum agar. Make up a 3 per cent. nutrient agar and tube in the ordinary way. Melt and cool to about 50° C. To each tube add half the quantity of sterile blood serum. Mix and pour into a petri dish. Incubate overnight to test sterility.

If glucose serum agar is required the nutrient agar should also contain 1 per cent. of glucose.

INDEX